TOUGH
CHOICES

TOUGH CHOICES

STORIES FROM THE FRONT LINE OF MEDICAL ETHICS

Daniel Sokol

The Book Guild Ltd

First published in Great Britain in 2018 by
The Book Guild Ltd
9 Priory Business Park
Wistow Road, Kibworth
Leicestershire, LE8 0RX
Freephone: 0800 999 2982
www.bookguild.co.uk
Email: info@bookguild.co.uk
Twitter: @bookguild

Typeset in Aldine401 BT

Printed and bound in Great Britain by CPI Group (UK) Ltd, Croydon, CR0 4YY

ISBN 978 1912575 480

British Library Cataloguing in Publication Data.
A catalogue record for this book is available from the British Library.

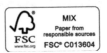

To Ella and Nicholas, my two delightful children, without whom this book would have been completed years ago

CONTENTS

CONTENTS

FOREWORD

Raanan Gillon
Emeritus Professor of Medical Ethics, Imperial College London

Before prefacing this fascinating collection of essays let me disclose an undoubted bias: Daniel has metamorphosed from PhD student showing signs of eternal student syndrome into my good friend as well as a star in the medical ethics and law firmament. There aren't many people with doctorates in medical ethics, a Masters in medical history, active participation in a wide range of clinical ethics contexts, and ongoing professional practice as a barrister specialising in medical law (not to mention continuing work as an award-winning medical journalist specialising in medical ethics and membership of the Magic Circle). So yes, I'm a great fan, and distinctly biased.

But I predict that many who read this collection of essays are also likely, if they aren't already members, to join the Sokol fan club, whether or not they agree with all his arguments and proposals. Thus even private surgeons carrying out entirely cosmetic vaginoplasty operations to create a 'designer vagina' should find his views engagingly thought-provoking (though perhaps also simply provoking.) And those of us who espouse the importance of empathy in the doctor–patient relationship may nonetheless find cause to reflect on what exactly we mean by empathy when we read Daniel's strictures and his preference for an Oslerian, kind but somewhat distant, imperturbability in his doctor.

Medical researchers who'd like to abolish research ethics committees should at least find themselves thinking again on reading 'Battling Professor Pinker'. And all of us will doubtless think again on reading his discomforting essays on 'doctors deceiving doctors' (his PhD was about deception) and on admitting error ('the hardest thing of all').

Polarised responses can also be expected to his support for decriminalisation of physician assisted suicide.

Altogether, Sokol addresses a huge range of ethics issues in this invigorating and fascinating collection of essays – a collection of ongoing relevance not only to doctors and other healthcare practitioners but also to all who are or might be at the other end of the stethoscope, i.e., most people!

Denigrating his own self-described 'foul-mouthed' behaviour after a footballing head injury (I blame the head injury) he reflects on the need for patient ethics as well as medical ethics. He warns against being inveigled by patients and others into behaviour that goes against the ethics of medicine. He argues that the reporting of medical unfitness to drive should be mandatory in the public interest, just as the reporting of many infectious diseases is mandatory even if patients request medical confidentiality or assure the doctor that they will self-report (after all, he points out, patients, for all sorts of understandable reasons of self-interest, may not fulfil that assurance and lives may be lost as a result).

Despite the brevity of the essays they are often packed with the nuances and complexities of issues in medical ethics. For example, the General Medical Council's 'make the care of your patient your first concern' is carefully unpacked into a rather more nuanced and accurate account of that bold instruction. Patients' relatives will be heartened by his plea to doctors: 'don't forget the relatives'. Sometimes the essays verge on the movingly poetical – see his ethicist in the neurology department and his perception of the 'essence of medicine'. At other times we are given down-to-earth lawyerly advice – the essays on the UK's Montgomery judgment on consent and on the basics of negligence law, for example.

I was particularly taken by the essay on 'the judge as ethicist'. Taking his cue from a case in which the parents of a 40-year-old man with an estimated mental age of 6-9 years and an IQ of 40 ask the court of protection to authorise a vasectomy in the man's best interests – I won't do a spoiler by going on with the story – Daniel points out the 'pedagogic' benefits of reading whole judgments rather than the brief extracts that are reported in the press and media. He praises the methodical analyses carried out by high court judges and contrasts this with some of the reasoning he has encountered in clinical contexts, including the reasoning in some ethics committees.

Let me also endorse Daniel's pleas for more medical ethicists to be employed in hospitals; it's a strange idea still to many UK doctors. (I recall the astonishment I felt in the '80s when I was touring medical ethics teaching establishments in the USA as one of my interviewees – a philosopher – was bleeped as we had coffee – the bleep was for an urgent clinical ethics consultation.) The fact is that clinical ethicists can be invaluable in helping clinicians deal with difficult realtime ethical problem cases.

Of course, there have to be caveats: clinical ethicists must have had exposure to real medical environments (something that Daniel himself has sought out from his earliest involvement with medical ethics – as comes through so clearly in this book but perhaps most poignantly in his story of Anastasia and the neurologist).

Clinical ethicists must also have common sense; a good knowledge of basic medical ethics and law; and, as Daniel advises, a basic knowledge and skill in the art of conflict resolution – so many of the actual day-to-day and night-to-night problems of medical ethics are inflamed by interpersonal conflict. In addition, clinical ethicists need to be available for advice and assistance when needed, 24 hours a day. Although some clinical ethics committees provide a facility for realtime ethics consultation, many do not. This is an area where the UK and indeed most of the rest of the world can learn a lesson from the USA.

One of the recurring themes in these essays is the special nature of medicine. Daniel criticises a philosopher for sneering at the 'solemn pledge' of service to humanity made in the latest version of the Declaration of Geneva, the World Medical Association's contemporary version of the Hippocratic oath. The philosopher had responded to the Declaration's 'I will foster the honour and noble traditions of the medical profession' by blogging "Huh? It's just a job, mate. Get over it."

Not at all says Daniel: 'Being a doctor is not just a job, or at least it should not be. It possesses a moral dimension not found in nearly all other jobs. Hence why there is no Professor in Baking Ethics, or Painting and Decorating Ethics, or Hairdressing Ethics... In the Hippocratic oath, the doctors swore by 'Apollo, Asclepius, Hygieia, Panacea and by all the gods and goddesses'. In the secular, modern-day version, doctors solemnly pledge. The purpose? To acknowledge the privilege, importance and dignity of treating a fellow human being in need.'

Hear hear, Daniel!

For me and no doubt for many medical readers of the *British Medical Journal* where Daniel has been 'Ethics Man' for many years, this is a dipping into sort of book but what a pleasurable educational and thought-provoking variety of dippings-in, dunkings and, for some, even total immersions it will provide.

PREFACE

This book represents nearly 15 years of thought on medical ethics and law.

Several of the chapters in this book first appeared, in modified form, as columns in the *British Medical Journal*. The readers of the *BMJ* are largely doctors and medical students. For this reason, and as many readers will be medically qualified, the book assumes a certain level of medical sophistication but none beyond the wit of the intelligent non-medic armed with the Internet, a medical dictionary or the glossary at the end of this book.

To my great fortune, the study and practice of medical ethics and law has taken me around the world, from Canada to New Zealand, via India and Hong Kong. I have worked as a clinical ethicist in opulent, state-of-the-art hospitals in the United States and volunteered in rural clinics with unreliable electricity in the poorer parts of India. I have advised government departments, Royal Colleges, multinational companies, and charities. I have encountered patients with remarkable stories and doctors both brilliant and appalling. As a barrister, I have represented clients of all sorts, from those with tetraplegia and other catastrophic injuries to those with lesser ills, such as the client whose faulty penile implant caused, to his great embarrassment, a permanent erection. Many of those stories have found their way into the pages of this book, although often anonymised.

The aim of this book is to present medical ethics and law in an accessible, engaging and relevant way to doctors and non-doctors alike. As we will all be patients at some stage in our lives, and may know loved ones who are or will be patients, medical ethics and law should be of practical interest and relevance to all. They should not only be the province of philosophers, doctors, or lawyers.

The chapters are grouped by themes, but each chapter is self-contained and can be read in isolation. The topics range from an analysis of individual cases, such as the Ashya King, Charlie Gard and Alfie Evans cases that gripped Britain in 2014, 2017, and 2018 respectively, to broader policy issues, such as the legalisation of assisted dying and the banning of boxing and other dangerous sports. If the answer to the problems and dilemmas cannot be found in the 800 words or so that make up each chapter, I hope at the very least to have set thought in motion.

I am grateful to the many people, too numerous to mention individually, who have helped and advised me over the years, including the patients who appear in these pages.

I must thank, however, Professor Jean Bernard (posthumously, as he died in 2006 at the age of 98) and Professor Raanan Gillon, who inspired me to study medical ethics. I am also grateful to my wife Sam, a consultant neurosurgeon, who from the outset acted as proofreader, medical consultant, and unforgiving critic. Any errors that somehow passed her fine filter remain mine alone.

London, May 2018

CHALLENGES IN THE DOCTOR–PATIENT RELATIONSHIP

THE HARMS OF MEDICOPLASTY

The 16th-century French author and doctor Rabelais was obsessed with vaginas. In one of his stories an old lady drives the devil away by showing him her vagina. Today the devil might recommend she go to the nearest aesthetic surgeon for vaginal rejuvenation. A touch off the labia (labiaplasty), a bit of tightening here (vaginoplasty), and voilà: a designer vagina.

The number of cosmetic genital operations is seemingly on the rise. The market for cosmetic procedures in the UK was £3.6 billion in 2015. In the United States, $20 billion. There are now lawyers specialising in negligence in cosmetic medicine. And yet, the market remains poorly regulated. According to the 2017 Nuffield Council Report on Cosmetic Procedures, "there are no controls on who may provide non-surgical procedures, other than limitations on access to prescription medicines, and on procedures in the mouth." Anyone can administer Botox or dermal fillers, for example.

The British Association of Aesthetic Plastic Surgeons, in its section on genital surgery, notes: "With a growing acceptance of surgery designed to alter appearance, and the increasing availability of explicit images of naked women, a number of women are requesting surgery to alter their intimate appearance, feeling that they compare unfavourably."

Here is my paternalistic view: medical professionals, whether working in the private or public sector, should not succumb to these requests. Although it would be hard to argue that anyone seeking aesthetic genital surgery is unable to make an informed decision, it is plausible to argue that patients' autonomy is often diminished by strong social or peer pressures. A female friend once told me how fat and ugly she felt after reading a popular women's magazine. She was neither fat nor ugly.

A drug company promoting a drug for hair loss – an issue close to my heart – urged balding men to consult their doctor. In a leading website on hair loss, sponsored by a drug company, a poll asks: "Have you felt less attractive since you started losing your hair?" Women seeking cosmetic genital surgery often bring pictures of their ideal vagina from advertisements or pornography.

Creating or exploiting insecurities is a lucrative business. Advertisements for cosmetic surgery are also manipulative, if not downright deceptive. How radiant and stunning the (digitally enhanced) models look! How easy and stress free the procedure is! The sheer number of advertisements and their wide exposure in public spaces suggest to passers-by that cosmetic surgery is not much different from a trip to the hairdresser.

In the eyes of the public, doctors are doctors, whether they practise in Harley Street or in an NHS hospital. Although aesthetic surgeons are a minority, their actions affect the image of the entire profession. Some genital operations, such as in vaginal prolapse or the reduction of grossly enlarged labia, are medically indicated; but if we extend the remit of medicine to capture requests for treatment on anatomically normal structures that have clear harm and uncertain benefit, the public's perception of doctors may suffer – all the more so if financial gain is involved. The public may lose trust because such procedures deviate from the spirit of the Hippocratic oath.

As medical science progresses, the oath retracts further into the communal consciousness of medicine, a distant star whose brightness is fading. Many medical students now know only its name. We should not let it fade, for it is the medical profession's guiding star. Although some parts of the oath are out of date, others contain unchanging truths: "I will use treatments for the benefit of the ill in accordance with my ability and my judgment, but from what is to their harm or injustice I will keep them." The key phrase is "for the benefit of the ill".

What constitutes an illness is not always easy to define (the philosopher Georges Canguilhem reflected on the changeable nature of the normal and the pathological decades ago), and grey areas exist, but a vagina that is not sufficiently tight according to the opinion of a partner or some pornographic ideal is no illness. The acquiescence of aesthetic surgeons, however, may help create a new illness.

In the transition from NHS to private doctor it is easy to slip, quite imperceptibly, into a more business-minded mode. The patient becomes a client, and the provider–client partnership may seem to differ from the doctor–patient relationship. In an act of self-deception we can lose sight of our conflict of interest and accede to the poorly thought out wishes of patients, dismissing the lure of money and hiding behind the convenient belief that it is the patient's autonomous choice: "If that's what they really want, and they understand the risks, then who am I to question it?"

The answer is: you are a doctor, not a tattoo artist. Committed to the Hippocratic ideal of treating the sick, doctors should not be complicit in the medicalisation of the normal by fulfilling the aesthetic desires of the worried well. Far from doing them good, they may let them down. Protecting patients – or keeping them from harm, in the words of the oath – may require persuading them that surgery is not the answer.

Today's doctors, like the Rabelaisian devil, should walk away from patients who ask for aesthetic genital surgery. Their wallets will be less full, but their integrity will remain. By altering the shape of women's normal labia and other similar procedures, doctors are altering the character of medicine.

Such medicoplasty has many risks and few benefits. Clinicians of all stripes, not just surgeons in the Hippocratic tradition, should speak out against "Hollywood" practitioners. The reputation of the medical profession, laboriously built up since physicians began to be university trained around the 13th century, is under threat.

MAKE THE CARE OF YOUR PATIENT YOUR FIRST CONCERN

The first rule of *Good Medical Practice*, a booklet issued by the General Medical Council to all doctors, is: "Make the care of your patient your first concern." The statement captures a fundamental truth about the practice of medicine, pointing to the sacred and timeless nature of the encounter between the healer and the sick person.

Yet, however noble in spirit, the rule should be no more than a rule of thumb. Although "patient" is in the singular, few doctors have only one patient. Doctors must therefore choose how to allocate their "concern" among their many patients. It is neither possible nor desirable to treat each patient as a first concern, as some patients, usually the sickest, merit more concern than others. The principle of justice requires the doctor to determine which patient deserves the greatest attention.

In a field hospital in a conflict zone, four patients are admitted after an explosion. One has multiple traumatic limb amputations. The others have less severe injuries but require blood transfusions. Treatment of the first victim will activate the massive transfusion protocol.

Should the hospital's entire stock of blood and plasma be used on that one patient? In such a situation triage priority shifts from "treat those in greatest medical need" to "save the most number of lives". The care of your multiple amputee is, regrettably, no longer your first concern. The rule is modified as follows: "Make the care of your patient your first concern, bearing in mind your other patients and their particular needs."

At times the interests of the public outweigh the obligation owed to an individual patient. A doctor is under an obligation to inform the authorities of a patient with yellow fever, however much the patient may protest. The first concern is not so much the patient but protecting the population from infection. So the revised rule is now: "Make the care of your patient your first concern, bearing in mind your other patients and their particular needs, as well as any protective obligations to the broader community."

A doctor's duty of care is not an absolute obligation, to be discharged however perilous the situation. In extreme circumstances – such as epidemics, where treating patients involves a high risk of infection and modest benefits to patients – doctors' obligations to their children, parents, siblings, and loved ones may take priority over the care of patients. The doctors who left their dying patients in the early outbreaks of Ebola haemorrhagic fever in Sudan and the Democratic Republic of Congo (in the late 1970s and 1980s) did not necessarily act unethically. The doctors and nurses who remained, many of whom lost their lives to the virus, acted beyond the call of duty.

The rule now looks as follows: "Make the care of your patient your first concern, bearing in mind your other patients and their particular needs, as well as any protective obligations to the broader community and obligations you may have towards others for whom you are responsible."

Even in ordinary times, making the care of your patient your first concern seems too demanding. A doctor's life, personal and professional, would be dominated by this over-riding concern; their working day would be interminably long, their holidays pitifully short. Their relations with friends, family, and others would suffer. They would not conduct research, publish articles, attend conferences, conduct activities that would further their career, or develop skills to help future patients, for the rule ignores their personal ambitions and talks only of the present patient.

The "bare" rule, strictly interpreted, would also pose problems for trainees learning to perform procedures. If a junior doctor is anxious about inserting a central line or removing a gall bladder, the rule suggests that he or she must ask a senior colleague to do it, as this is probably best for that particular patient. A trainee is more likely than an experienced colleague to make a mistake or cause discomfort, even if supervised. Yet this logic is not conducive to learning and development. Although the present patient will benefit, future patients will suffer.

Thus the updated rule is: "In your professional capacity as a doctor, make the care of your patient your first concern, bearing in mind your other patients, including at times future patients, and their particular needs as well as any protective obligations to the broader community, your own obligations to develop your skills and knowledge as a clinician, and obligations you may have towards others for whom you are responsible."

Finally, the rule can be misused. I have heard doctors invoke the rule to justify their exaggerations to radiologists to expedite their patient's scans. Doctors in the United States have been known to deceive insurance companies to obtain treatments for their patients. If the care of your patient is your first concern, this may lead you to flout other rules, including legal ones.

So the final version of the rule is: "In your professional capacity as a doctor, make the care of your patient your first concern, acting within morally and legally acceptable limits and bearing in mind your other patients, including at times future patients and their particular needs as well as any protective obligations to the broader community, your own obligations to develop your skills and knowledge as a clinician, and obligations you may have towards others for whom you are responsible."

The first rule of the GMC is a profoundly important statement, but its brevity necessarily obscures the complexity of modern medical practice. Ironically, too literal a reading of the rule could lead to unethical conduct. It should be seen as a starting point, not a commandment.

BEWARE THE LIES OF PATIENTS

In 2003, I started a PhD in Medical Ethics. I took great pride in the simplicity of my research question, which was reducible to eight words: "Should doctors always tell the truth to patients?" The answer, after three years of hard labour, was "most of the time". The other 99,000 words merely elaborated on that answer, but there was one digression that examined how patients deceive doctors.

This fascinating and understudied issue appears in the Hippocratic corpus in the 4th and 5th centuries BC. One passage advises readers to "keep a watch also on the faults of the patients, which often make them lie about the taking of things prescribed."

In the early 1990s Burgoon and colleagues reported that 85% of the patients they interviewed admitted concealing or equivocating about information to their doctors, and roughly a third claimed to have lied to their doctors.

Patients deceive doctors for various reasons. With some patients, the deception forms part of their attempt to assume a 'sick role', as in factitious disorders such as Münchausen's syndrome (where the mentally ill patient pretends to be sick). Other patients deceive to get disability benefits, to maximise damages in personal injury litigation, to avoid a sojourn in prison, or, in countries with mandatory military service, to evade conscription.

Some patients deceive to enjoy the shelter, warmth, and food of the hospital. One doctor told me of a homeless patient in his hospital's emergency department who claimed to have no sensation in his legs but who jumped up in agony when pricked with a pin.

Some patients feign ignorance to obtain an independent second opinion or even to 'test' the knowledge of an unfamiliar doctor.

In my work as a barrister, I regularly read medicolegal reports about patients with whiplash injuries sustained in road traffic crashes. Some of these reports detail injuries that seem grossly disproportionate to the violence of the impact. One senior member of the insurance industry told me that some doctors are flown in from abroad to examine patients one after the other in a cheap hotel room and draft brief medicolegal reports on a pro forma document before returning to their country of origin.

In a recent trial of mine, the injured client told the judge that he had only spent 5 minutes with the GP who allegedly examined him thoroughly and produced the 10-page report for the court. There is little doubt that some of these medical 'experts', who can write thousands of reports a year (at £180 each), are complicit in the lies of patients told to insurance companies.

GPs will know of patients who claimed that they could not bend their back but effortlessly picked up a magazine from the low table in the surgery's waiting room or those who averred that they could barely walk without excruciating pain but could be seen outside ambling in apparent comfort. Some patients present with unexplained pain and insist that only strong opioids can soothe the pain. These patients join online groups giving tips on ways to get the desired drug. When the GP or other staff explore non-opioid alternatives, the patients may not be interested.

Doctors are advocates for patients. They must act in the best interests of their patients and respect their autonomy. Yet these are not absolute injunctions. Doctors are moral agents whose autonomy is also deserving of respect. Complying with the requests of patients must not undermine clinicians' moral and professional integrity. If a request requires the doctor to act in a manner that is morally wrong (such as making them complicit in fraud) or not medically indicated, then the doctor should politely decline.

Barristers are occasionally asked to make arguments by the lay client or the client's solicitors that they believe are hopeless. Only last week I was asked by a solicitor to persuade a judge to award the cost of an item that, in law, was plainly irrecoverable. "Give it a go," the solicitor said. The Bar Code of Conduct states that a barrister "must not make a submission [in court] which he does not consider to be properly arguable." The same principle should apply to doctors: their actions must, from a medical perspective, be properly arguable. If doctors could not defend their action, or omission, to a group of peers, then they should turn down the patient's request and suggest a second opinion.

The manner in which this is done is important. It should be without a hint of reproach. In some cases, however, the relationship will be irretrievably damaged, however diplomatic and sensitive the doctor's language.

It is true that complicity in the deception may be the easier option (at least in the short term), avoiding a potentially long and awkward discussion. Sadly, however, doing the right thing is sometimes more onerous than the alternatives.

THE LIMITS OF CONFIDENTIALITY

Poppy-Arabella was 3 years old. On 6th July 2016 she and her mother were on their way to nursery. As they crossed a road at a red traffic light, a car approached. It did not slow down or swerve, and it struck them both in the middle of the crossing. Poppy-Arabella was killed; her mother was seriously injured.

The driver, John Place, was 72. He had poor eyesight and did not see the red light, the crossing, or the pedestrians. He just heard a scream, a thump, and the sound of his windscreen shattering.

Three weeks earlier, two optometrists had told Mr Place to stop driving. He pleaded guilty to causing death by dangerous driving and was sentenced to four years in prison. This case raises the familiar question about medical secrecy: should healthcare professionals breach confidentiality when a patient is unfit to drive?

The General Medical Council (GMC) has guidance on reporting concerns to the Driver and Vehicle Licensing Agency (DVLA). Doctors should explain to patients deemed unfit to drive that their condition may affect their ability to drive and that they – the patients – have a legal obligation to inform the DVLA about their condition.

If the patient continues to drive, the GMC advises that "you should make every reasonable effort to persuade them to stop." If persuasion fails or the doctor discovers that the patient is continuing to drive, the doctor should contact the DVLA to disclose the medical information.

The trouble with this approach is that it relies on patients' honesty. Many patients will lie to avoid the loss of their driving licence. Unable to drive, they may no longer be able to get to work. They may not be able to collect their children. They may need to take taxis at great expense. With much to lose, they will falsely promise to inform the DVLA and to stop driving. And the chances of the doctor discovering that the patient is continuing to drive are slim.

Motor vehicles are lethal objects. They maim and kill innocent people just as efficiently as infectious diseases or terrorist attacks. Doctors in the public interest are required by law to report patients who have certain infectious diseases or who may commit terrorist acts – but strangely not patients who may cause serious harm through their unfitness to drive.

Logic calls for the law of disclosure to extend to patients deemed unfit to drive or fly. The GMC should consider making disclosure to the DVLA mandatory, even if the patient confirms that this has been or will be done. To rely on the assurances of patients, in the knowledge that they – like most of us – lie to please others and to get out of trouble, is naive and irresponsible. It can also cost lives.

Poppy-Arabella's parents are calling for this strict

disclosure policy to become law. Such a policy may dissuade patients from disclosing information that they would otherwise reveal if secrecy was guaranteed. Yet secrecy is not guaranteed at present: it can be breached if the patient refuses to discharge his or her legal obligation to inform the DVLA or if the doctor discovers that the patient is still driving. The difference is that doctors would no longer rely on the unverified promises of the patient. They would automatically tell the DVLA that the patient was unfit to drive.

This new law would not erode doctor–patient confidentiality. It offers a solution to the reluctance of impaired drivers to acknowledge the danger they pose to others, as well as the recognition that some patients will deceive to continue driving.

DON'T FORGET THE RELATIVES

The 25-year-old patient had a rare skin disorder called Stevens-Johnson syndrome. She had been in intensive care for several days. One morning, at 9.40 am, her core temperature was 38.5°C. At 10 am it had climbed to 40.5°C. By 1.30 pm it was 42°C. At 4 pm it had risen to 43°C. It reached 44.4°C before she went into cardiac arrest. After 10 cycles of cardiopulmonary resuscitation she was pronounced dead, at 6.13 pm.

Nine months later I represented the patient's relatives at the inquest. They said they had no idea she might die, that no one had bothered to tell them quite how sick she was. "If we had known," the mother said, "we would have stayed with her in that room the whole time." Their complaint is a familiar one.

Historically, the clinician's gaze has been focused on the patient. The patient's intimates have remained in the shadows. The doctor–patient dyad leaves out the family, and there is no mention of the sick person's relatives in the Hippocratic oath.

Confidentiality, or keeping the secrets of patients, places limits on the extent of the family's involvement. If a patient has capacity, the clinician should check that sharing information with relatives is permitted. If the patient lacks capacity, the GMC's guidance reflects the commonsense position: "It is reasonable to assume that, unless they indicate otherwise, they would want those closest to them to be kept informed of relevant information about their general condition and prognosis."

When a patient is ill, clinicians consider whether that patient knows the diagnosis and prognosis. If not, and if the patient has capacity, the norm in the United Kingdom, the United States, and many other countries is to disclose that information to the patient. Respect for patient autonomy requires it. Yet, clinicians should also consider whether the relatives should be told about the patient's condition.

The family of the patient in my inquest wanted regular updates. They believed that the patient was stable until a junior doctor rushed to the hospital cafeteria to tell them that she had gone into cardiac arrest. Although the family believed that there was a sudden and catastrophic turn for the worse, the medical notes show a gradual decline over hours. The clinicians suspected she might die. The relatives were clueless.

Talking to the family ranks low in a clinician's list of priorities. In busy times, dealing with other patients may push that task so low on the list that it never gets done on that shift. After checking the patient's observations, noting urine output, calculating fluid balance, reading scans, arranging for tests, phoning colleagues, and conducting other tasks, a doctor may forget to talk to the family. Sharing bad news can also be an unpleasant task for clinicians. Some relatives ask irritating questions, others complain about the patient's management or talk too much, and others are downright rude.

Time is a limited resource in medicine, but keeping relatives informed of the patient's condition is time well spent. Regular discussions set the family's expectations at the right level. They reduce the likelihood of conflict arising from divergent understandings of the patient's true condition. They build trust, show concern, and reflect an appreciation that illness affects not just the patient but can "infect" their loved ones too, causing emotional pain and suffering. They can allow relatives to explain the medical situation to the patient in more meaningful ways or help persuade the patient to follow a course of action. And when patients lose capacity relatives can form valuable allies in making decisions that reflect the patient's values.

When the patient is in pain or appears distressed, it is particularly important to explain the situation to the family, including the steps taken to minimise the distress. At the inquest the relatives could not understand why the patient had struggled to breathe when the anaesthetist could have used the ventilator to breathe for her. It was an upsetting sight. In fact, the anaesthetist wanted to exercise the patient's ailing lungs, but this was never explained to the relatives, who instead believed that the medical team had neglected her. More than any other, the sight of a patient in distress, without any explanation for that distress or reassurance that everything has been done to keep the patient comfortable, can lead relatives to question the quality of care provided. This, in turn, increases the likelihood of complaints.

So accustomed are clinicians to treating sick patients that some barely notice the relatives standing helplessly by the bedside and forget what William Osler reminded the nurses at the Philadelphia Hospital in 1897: "The handing over to a stranger the care of a life precious beyond all computation may be one of the greatest earthly trials." Keeping the relatives informed of the medical situation, good or bad, makes the ordeal more bearable.

If we are the relatives and feel poorly informed about the care of our loved one, then we must be proactive in our quest for information and ask – courteously of course – for an update, however busy the medical staff may appear and whatever the risk of causing irritation. Without such an approach, we will probably remain at the bottom of the doctor's "to do" list.

HIPPOCRATES, MICHAEL JACKSON AND MEDICAL ETHICS

The Hippocratic oath has a part where the action shifts from the public sphere to the private: "Into as many houses as I may enter I will go for the benefit of the ill." After the death of Michael Jackson in June 2009, at age 50, suspicious eyes turned towards the singer's personal physician, Conrad Murray. Dr Murray was convicted for involuntary manslaughter in November 2011 and sentenced to 4 years in prison.

The incident forced the doctor–patient relationship into the spotlight. How does the dynamic of this relationship alter when the patient is more powerful than the doctor?

In medical school we teach students to be aware of the power differential between doctor and patient. In a hospital setting, patients may be sick, frightened, and medically unsophisticated. Doctors, on the other hand, are generally healthy, medically knowledgeable, and in a familiar environment. Such is the typical clinical encounter. Doctors are strong; patients are vulnerable. In some cases, however, the power relationship is altered and a different set of challenges arises.

At times the locus of power is external. Military

doctors, for example, can be both physicians and soldiers. They have superiors whose orders they must obey and for whom the welfare of a patient may be less important than the military mission. Edmund Howe, a psychiatrist who served in the US army, gives the example of treating patients with combat fatigue in the battlefield. If a military psychiatrist allows a soldier with combat fatigue to return home, many more soldiers may feign symptoms to escape combat. This floodgate effect may undermine the mission's success. The doctor's dual loyalty to the military and to patients is an example of mixed agency.

Mixed agency also exists in the field of sports medicine. Sports doctors may be torn between their duties to the patient and their duties, as an employee of the club, to the manager. Should a star athlete with an injury be allowed to compete if the manager instructs the club doctor that he or she should? An injection of painkillers will satisfy the manager and may improve the team's performance, but the patient will be put at risk. As these are coveted medical jobs, the manager would have no trouble finding a replacement.

Should self-interest trump the lofty principles of medical ethics? Should the scope of best interests be enlarged to encompass the team? As in the military situation, the manager has the best interests of the team in mind, and this will not always coincide with the medical best interests of the patient.

In April 2009, in the quarter final of rugby's Heineken Cup, the club doctor of the Harlequins team deliberately cut a player's lip, at the player's request, so that a specialist goal kicker could be brought on. The player had concealed a capsule of fake blood in his sock. In causing physical harm to the patient, the doctor had put the team's interests over that of her patient, and over the laws and spirit of the sport. She was suspended by the GMC.

A sports doctor once told me that he allowed a boxer, ahead on points in the biggest fight of his life, to continue fighting with a broken rib. The tension here was between the medical best interests of the patient (stop the fight) and his overall best interests (allow him to fulfil his ambition of reaching the top of the sport).

One notable area where the power differential is reversed is in the medical care of heads of state. When in office François Mitterrand, who was the French president from 1981 to 1995, told his personal physician, Claude Gubler, that his diagnosis of prostate cancer was a "state secret" that should be kept even from the president's wife. For the next 11 years Dr Gubler prepared and signed medical bulletins giving the president a clean bill of health and never mentioning his cancer. When laboratory tests were needed Dr Gubler sent specimens under a pseudonym. Meanwhile Mitterrand justified his pains by disguising them as tennis injuries.

France is a nuclear power, and it seems reasonable that someone should know if the president, who can pull the nuclear trigger, has experienced a decline in mental competence, succumbed to a drug or alcohol addiction, or is simply spending all of his time in bed, as was the case with Mitterrand towards the end of 1994. Keeping a medical secret is not an absolute obligation, but breaching confidentiality must be particularly challenging when your patient is a president or prime minister.

As personal physicians tend to spend prolonged periods with their patients – in times of sickness and, significantly, of health – a danger exists that professional boundaries become blurred and judgment impaired. The prestige of the job and a generous salary can also distort ethical and clinical judgment. For the unscrupulous and unreflective doctor, life can be sweet.

For the more thoughtful ones, knowingly practising ethically dubious medicine can be emotionally distressing. The Hippocratic oath was written at a time when doctors were not the trusted professionals they are today. Medicine was unregulated, and charlatans abounded. Such was the potential for abuse that the author of the oath stressed the need for moral and professional integrity: "In a pure and holy way, I will guard my life and my art and my science."

For private doctors of the 21st century, the public's trust in the profession, external pressure from third parties, the social power of some patients, relative isolation from colleagues, and the temptations of money, fame, and luxury combine to create barriers to good practice. These barriers are not, I think, insurmountable, but they must firstly be recognised.

Education at undergraduate and postgraduate level about the challenges of caring for powerful patients, of mixed agency, and of self-interest may go some way towards revealing the barriers. However, no amount of education and no code of practice will resolve all the ethical problems. When the moment of truth comes, only individual doctors can decide whether to choose their art, their ego, or their pocket.

HOW (NOT) TO BE A GOOD PATIENT

One Saturday in February 2004, as I leapt in the air,
salmon-like, to head the winning goal for the local
football team, a clumsy defender bashed his head
against mine. The impact of his forehead created such
a deep, unsightly dent over my right eye that the other
players, visibly repulsed by the wound, called for an
ambulance.

When the ambulance finally arrived, several
interminable minutes past the government's eight-
minute target, the two paramedics waltzed in, sprightly
and cheerful, in their green and yellow overalls. I was
bothered by their apparent indifference to my plight –
the alarming possibility of death or of life as a vegetable
– but I mustered the inner strength to answer their
questions: "How did it happen?" "Where were you hit?"
"Where does it hurt?" and so on.

I was trolleyed into the ambulance and taken to the
hospital. The ambulance did not howl on the way there,
which angered me further. Was my potentially life-
threatening injury not serious enough to warrant the
howler?

In the emergency room a nurse asked me how I'd
been injured, where I was at the time, where it hurt, and

so on. She then left me in the middle of the room, still in my wheelchair and holding the now melted ice pack on my demolished forehead, for 20 minutes. Doctors and nurses walked past without so much as a glance. I felt totally abandoned. "What the fuck is going on?" I eventually exclaimed, desperate to catch somebody's attention.

A sombre nurse emerged from a cubicle and told me not to swear. I apologised, blaming my foul mood on the injury. She pushed the wheelchair into the vacant cubicle and started a familiar interrogation: "How did it happen?" "Where were you hit?" "Where does it hurt?" and so on. I answered the questions as before. "The doctor's on his way," she told me as she left.

It looked as though the doctor was going to take an even longer time to appear than the paramedics had. When I questioned the nurse about the delay, she replied, "He won't be a minute." Ten minutes later there was still no sign of the doctor. As the pain grew worse I started whining.

A young doctor eventually arrived, apologised profusely for the wait, and injected me with painkillers. He then asked me how I'd injured my head, where the impact had occurred, where it hurt, and so on. Suppressing a mounting sense of frustration I answered the questions exactly as before, unable to understand the need for a fourth account of the incident. Throughout the whole ordeal I was undeniably grumpy, foul-mouthed, and ill-tempered. When I returned home that evening it dawned on me that being a patient – a good patient – must be terribly difficult.

People often discuss what makes a good or bad doctor. A good doctor, for example, must be knowledgeable, technically adept, compassionate, patient, kind, trustworthy, morally sound, and a great communicator. But how often do we hear of the good patient? Hardly ever. The good patient is the unsung hero of the clinic.

There is a striking similarity between the virtues of the good doctor and those of the good patient. Good patients are at once compassionate towards fellow patients and overworked hospital staff, tolerant when awaiting their turn and answering oft repeated questions, kind when communicating with others, trustworthy when reporting facts or taking their medicine, and, above all, understanding of the limitations and fallibility of medicine. I failed in nearly all of these counts. Whereas the good doctor must exercise these virtues and qualities while under pressure from bickering patients, anxious relatives, and limited time, the good patient must apply them in times of physical or emotional pain.

As patients we should strive to emulate those who suffer with such noble deportment and deplore those who, like me, disregard the interests of others as soon as the going gets a little tough. Diderot, the 18th-century French author, called poverty and disease "those two great exorcists". In other words a person's true nature is revealed not when that person is eating grapes and sipping champagne in a marbled jacuzzi but when under the stress of misery and ill health. At such times all that remains is a person's very core, devoid of pretence and superficiality.

The good patient, then, embodies the most genuine type of human goodness. My brief but dishonourable stint in hospital convinced me that patients deserve as much praise and criticism for their behaviour as doctors and that the public should be educated on the proper conduct in the stressful environment of the hospital.

PATIENTS WE DON'T LIKE

A few years ago, I was the barrister for a man who had been involved in a road traffic accident. Shortly before the trial we discussed – in private – what had happened on that day.

During the trial, it became evident during the course of cross-examination that my client was lying. There was video footage (unseen by me before the day of the trial) to confirm it. He had also breached my trust and lied to me repeatedly. Not a white lie, or a slight inaccuracy, but whopping great untruths.

With each passing minute, as his credibility floundered, my resolve to win the case weakened. I grew emotionally more distant from my client. By the end of the cross-examination I was filled with a profound dislike for him. It was an unsettling experience.

The trial was not over. In my closing submissions I still had to persuade the judge that my client was not negligent.

Similar situations arise in medicine. Until medicine is performed by robots, emotions will always feature in practice. Patients who are rude, angry, abusive, malodorous, self-destructive, time-wasters, or non-compliant and bed-blocking can arouse negative emotions in the treating clinician, especially when he or she is tired. These emotions, in turn, can lead to a lower standard of care for these "problem" patients.

The late Richard Selzer was that rare combination of surgeon and writer. In his essay *Brute* a surgeon has to suture a deep wound on a drunken, violent, and enraged patient's forehead at 2.45 am. When the surgeon asks him to hold still, the patient retorts, "You fuckin' hold still." Furious and exhausted, the surgeon sutures the patient's ears to the mattress of the stretcher, pinning his head still, then leans in to the patient and whispers, "Now you fuckin' hold still."

While saints can feel compassion, empathy, and love for the most loathsome of patients, and construct scenarios in which patients' bad behaviour is explained by difficult circumstances, to mere mortals such patients are, at best, unpleasant to endure. In these circumstances the doctor–patient relationship is strained.

Teachers of medical ethics will know that many medical students, and some clinicians, believe there to be no right or wrong answers in ethics. Ethics, they say, is merely a matter of opinion. This is a situation where the answer to the ethical question is clear. Under the GMC's *Duties of a Doctor*, doctors should "make the care of your patient your first concern" however odious the patient may be. Doctors should never discriminate unfairly against patients. The ethical principles of beneficence (doing good) and non-maleficence (not doing harm) underpin the guidance. The principle of justice also requires the fair treatment of patients, in accordance with their human rights.

Similarly, in the moments before making my closing submissions in the trial of my lying client, I remembered the Bar *Code of Conduct*, which states that barristers "must promote and protect fearlessly... the lay client's best interests."

In addition to the underlying ethical tensions, such cases are psychologically stressful. In an attempt to put my negative emotions aside, I recalled John Mortimer's instruction that barristers should cultivate lucid indifference. And so, buoyed by the demands of professionalism, I stood on my hind legs and delivered an impassioned speech on why my client should win. While I hoped that my body language revealed nothing of my inner doubts, in my heart of hearts I did not believe one word of my speech. Thankfully, neither did the judge. He found in favour of the other side.

Doctors are susceptible to making moral evaluations of their patients, but they should not let those evaluations adversely affect their treatment of their patients' illnesses. Like barristers in court, they are not judges of right and wrong. Their role is primarily focused on treating the sick. Like actors, they should show nothing of their displeasure. There should be no disapproving look or frown or words. Expression of any moral judgment should be suppressed.

This ability to provide expert services dispassionately to all patients and clients lies at the heart of professionalism. For those of us who are not saintly, this may involve the biting of tongues and, literally, "acting" professionally. When dealing in a professional capacity with people we dislike, perhaps lucid indifference and professional concern are more realistic goals than full-blown compassion.

It is important to recognise in ourselves the feelings of dislike, when they do arise. Unless we do we cannot consciously manage them and reduce the likelihood of bias. Our more brutish instincts may take over, and our profession, reputation, self-respect, and patients may suffer.

CULTURE, SOCIETY AND MEDICINE

A VOYAGE TO INDIA

In June 2007, I was invited to lecture to a group of doctors in a hospital in Stoke-on-Trent. The topics were informed consent and truth-telling, and I stressed the importance of respecting patients' wishes, even if they clashed with our own, and reminded my audience to consider when, where, and how to tell the truth. Disclosing a grim truth at the wrong time or in too blunt a manner can be harmful to patients and their relatives.

Two weeks later, after an 11-hour plane journey and a perilous 6-hour taxi ride, I arrived in the Indian state of Tamil Nadu where, for the next month, I would be observing the work of a rural surgeon. In the morning, the surgeon acted as a surgically-trained GP, seeing patients as they walked in from the street. He drained abscesses, cleaned wounds, checked orifices, and treated infections of all sorts. The afternoon was devoted to surgery. An appendix was removed here, a uterus there, haemorrhoids sliced off, a hernia repaired, a gaping wound stitched up. The 20 or so rooms in the hospital were small, basic, and crowded.

In some rooms, every inch of space was filled by relatives, sometimes as many as 10, sitting on the floor. The ceiling fan could do little against the flies and the sweltering heat. After my hair-raising car journey from the airport, I was not surprised to find many of the rooms occupied by victims of road traffic accidents. Those that were not were usually inhabited by diabetic patients, too often with wounds so large and deep that the muscles and bones were exposed below.

In one of the rooms was Rajendran, an elderly diabetic man, with a bandaged foot leaking brown fluid. His foot was so gangrenous that it could not be saved. To have any chance of survival, he had to undergo an above-knee amputation.

The next day, I helped hoist Rajendran onto the operating table. He was scared, muttering quietly to himself as the spinal anaesthetic was administered. The surgeon made a deep incision above the left knee and cut away through the fat and muscles until he reached the bone. The bone was cut using what looked like a cheese wire. After a few more strokes with the scalpel, a nurse lifted the severed leg from the table and dumped the heavy object in a plastic bowl.

The following day, the surgeon and I were driving to nearby villages to fix a perforated ulcer in a young man's intestines and to stitch up a lady's poorly closed caesarean wound. As we overtook an elephant on a truck, he told me Rajendran was unaware of the amputation. When he first suggested the procedure, Rajendran refused. The poor prognosis without surgery – another month or so of life – did not change his mind. So his family told him that the surgeon would simply fix his thigh. This, they said, would allow the blood to flow once again to his foot. Rajendran had reluctantly agreed.

Three days after the operation, Rajendran still did not know the truth. Although he noticed his lower leg was missing, he believed it would be reattached once the wound healed. As the junior doctor told me on my first morning at the hospital, most patients knew nothing about medicine.

This ignorance in matters medical, as well as the consultation fee of 50 rupees (roughly 75p), is partly why patients seek medical help much later than in the UK. One day, a 70-year-old woman walked in with an advanced carcinoma of the uterus. The prognosis was bleak. For the previous 6 months, some of her relatives had encouraged her to see a doctor but she had waved off their concerns, saying she would get better at home. That same day, a 60-year-old man sat next to the surgeon and whispered a few words in his ear, smiling nervously. Since his circumcision 20 years ago, something was not quite right down below.

When he removed his underwear, the tip of his penis was missing and the remaining tissue was covered in tarry craters, like miniature volcanoes covered in soot. To treat the carcinoma, the surgeon would have to remove the penis and the scrotum. It was only because the craters blocked his urethra and affected his peeing that he visited the doctor. For some patients, a small growth was one that could barely be seen a mile away.

In the UK, the ethical principle of respect for patient autonomy prohibits deception. Competent adults can refuse any procedure, however life-threatening and for whatever reason. When working as a clinical ethicist, I once came across a young man who was admitted to hospital with a perforated bowel. He was otherwise in good health. When invited to consent for life-saving surgery, he declined all treatment without giving reasons for his refusal. No amount of persuasion, from the medical team or his relatives, could change his mind. Deemed competent by psychiatrists, he was allowed to die.

In this corner of India, patient autonomy could be trumped by the autonomous wishes of the family. There was a strong spirit of community and family responsibility at odds with the Western focus on individual choice. The surgeon was certain that Rajendran would come to accept his relatives' decision.

Doctors are highly respected figures in India. A 10-year-old boy wore a T-shirt which read "future doctor". A letter from an X-ray lab to the surgeon started with "Respected doctor". Patients are submissive and the paternalistic dictum 'doctor knows best' prevails. I am still shocked by the surgeon's angry outbursts. One morning, a 22-year-old man entered the consultation room. After a brief exchange, the surgeon asked the female junior doctor and the nurses to leave the room: a tell-tale sign that the problem was located in an intimate area.

The patient pulled down his underwear and laid face down on the bed while the surgeon pushed a hollow metal instrument – a proctoscope – deep in his rectum.

The patient winced in pain. The surgeon shouted at him, slapping his buttocks and telling him to stop clenching. "Look," he told me, "can you see the change in colour?" Down the proctoscope, the pink mucosa turned a darker red. The patient had haemorrhoids.

As I reflect on these events, I smile at the thought of the surgeon and his nurses attending my earlier lecture in Stoke-on-Trent. No doubt they would have been bemused and concerned by our obsession with respecting patients' choices, however foolish these may appear.

Walking down a busy road in the small town challenged many of the senses. The ears were deafened by the incessant horns of swerving cars, rickshaws, and motorbikes. The nose was offended by exhaust fumes or some stench from the garbage strewn about the street. When the dust spared the eyes, they could feast on roaming pigs, goats, cows, stray dogs, myriad food stands swarmed by flies, and of course hundreds of people going about their lives ("India lives in its villages," Gandhi once observed).

To the consternation of doctors, many people wandered about barefoot, inviting abscesses to develop and parasitic worms to enter the body from below. If you looked carefully and for long enough, you would see a few people defecating on the side of the road. Many homes did not have toilets. A simple stroll there was an experience to behold. Exhilarating, surprising, exhausting.

After examining a man's genitals, the surgeon

provided the understatement of the trip: "Some of our people, their personal hygiene is not so good". Fungal infections and gastroenteritis were common and, due to the sheer number of people living in close proximity, so were respiratory infections. Poor hygiene goes hand in hand with poverty.

In a government hospital I visited, a 3-year-old child lay still on a hospital bed, his legs as thin as matchsticks. His story was a familiar one. The youngest of 6 children, the family did not have the resources to feed him properly, preferring to focus their attention on the older siblings. Of all India's health problems, malnutrition ranks as one of the most serious. The 2017 *Global Hunger Index* report ranked India 100 out of 119 countries, placing it at the upper end of the 'serious' category. Tamil Nadu is one of the worst affected states in India.

Some of the doctors I met attributed the ill health to the low literacy level in Tamil Nadu (a little over 80%) which, although pitiful by European standards, fared well for India. If you flicked through the one-page consent forms in the hospital, every so often you would find, in the 'signature' box, a fingerprint representing the digital evidence of illiterate patients. The thought was that uneducated patients were difficult to treat due to their limited understanding of medicine, their poor hygiene habits, and their low compliance. When I expressed my surprise at the harsh treatment of some patients, a doctor told me that without such a direct approach the message would never get through to "such people".

I could not help but feel, however, that this was not the whole story. Patients from the lower socio-economic classes were sometimes treated in ways that would be unthinkable in the UK or North America. Angry words, rough handling, and general neglect were all too common. In the consultation room and operating theatre, maintaining patient comfort and dignity were low on the list of priorities. The power differential between doctors and patients was such that few patients would express their discontent. Indeed, many expected such treatment. While I admired the technical virtuosity of the doctors and surgeons I met here, I felt the human dimension of patient care could be greatly improved. Care and functionality could coexist.

A caring approach was a taller order in government hospitals, where the average consultation lasted about 30 seconds. Government hospitals were free and the domain of the poorest. Each day, 900 or so outpatients stood in line for a 'consultation', the men in one line, the women in another. Physical examinations were the exception rather than the rule. The normal routine in the 30 seconds consisted of a glance at the problem area, the medical history, a few scribbles on a notepad, and a wave to indicate the next patient's turn. "What do British doctors do for 8 minutes?" asked a puzzled doctor when I told him of the average consultation time in the UK in 2007. It is now 8-10 minutes.

In rural areas, the challenges of ill health were made worse by inadequate medical facilities. One week, in different villages, a power cut disabled the overhead operating lights during a surgery, the surgeon's headlights stopped working during a tonsillectomy (requiring me to shine a torch down the poor boy's throat), the suction pump draining the blood got blocked during a messy caesarean section, and several surgeries were performed without that most sought-after of doctors, the anaesthetist. "Indian surgeons can cope with anything," said the surgeon after removing tonsils in semi-darkness. The world-class facilities of some large Indian cities seemed a million miles away.

If you want fast service and technical excellence, go to southern Tamil Nadu and you can have your operation done that very day for a most reasonable price. A hysterectomy (surgical removal of the uterus), for example, will cost you £200, all inclusive, and a hernia repair a modest £120 with 5-day hospital accommodation. Be warned however that the post-operative hospital stay is no sojourn at the Hilton. If you want to guarantee respectful, compassionate treatment, an anaesthetist at the bedside, a blood transfusion if something goes wrong, a modicum of comfort, and good operating conditions for the surgeon, then this corner of rural India is not for you.

In the weeks after the operation to amputate his leg, Rajendran held different beliefs about his missing leg.

He first believed that the severed portion would be reattached once the operative wound had healed. Later, the surgeon told him that a 'walking implement' would be fitted to his stump. Still later, he suffered from phantom limb syndrome and believed his leg to be whole, sometimes gingerly feeling the vacant area beyond the stump.

One Wednesday, the surgeon told him the truth. I was curious to see how Rajendran would react. The surgeon revealed the well-intentioned deception and explained the reasoning behind it. An exchange between the surgeon and patient ensued, which ended in Rajendran shaking the surgeon's hand. "You see," said the surgeon, "he told me a doctor would only do what's best for him. He's happy."

That evening, I asked two nurses if Rajendran was satisfied. "No," answered one, "he's angry at his wife and sons for having lied to him." Was the deception justified? Without it, Rajendran would probably have died in a matter of weeks. Is this reason enough to violate his autonomy? This is no ethics lecture. You can draw your own conclusions.

Dozens of patients came and went in the days that followed. A young girl arrived in the hospital, holding an X-ray showing the cotton-like appearance of tuberculous lungs. As part of a government eradication programme, she received the drugs at no cost. The condition was so common that the local government hospital had a separate TB ward. In England, there are about 6,000 cases of TB per year; in India, 2.2 million.

One elderly man shuffled into the consultation room with six boils around the circumference of his head. The largest one, on his forehead, gave him the appearance of a human unicorn. The surgeon told him to donate his hair to the Hindu gods. This would also clear the way for a proper look. Twenty minutes later, the patient returned with a shaved scalp. The surgeon inserted scissors into each boil, forming craters which oozed rivulets of pus and blood. The pain was such that I held the patient's kicking feet. "Should we not give some anaesthetic?" I asked. "Only if he says it's intolerable," came the answer.

A crying 8-year-old boy arrived with a finger split in two. He'd got it caught in a water pump as his mother was drawing water. Again, in the consultation room itself, the dangling halves were stitched up there and then. This was medicine as magic. That afternoon, a 40-year-old woman was on a hospital bed with an enormous abdomen. Her spleen was, in the language of the lab report, 'massive'. The monster was removed that very day and she returned to her hospital bed with a deflated abdomen.

Other cases took longer to heal. A young chef at a nearby restaurant arrived with extensive burns on his face, chest, and left arm, the victim of a toppled pan of boiling oil. Recovery would be slow and his damaged eyes could require new corneas.

In one bed, a middle-aged lady, plagued by family problems, had attempted suicide by dousing herself in kerosene and setting herself ablaze, while another patient, a pretty 17-year-old girl with the same intent, had ingested liberal amounts of insecticide following a quarrel at school. The young girl spent a month in a coma. I asked the surgeon if after 20 years of practice anything still shocked him. "No," he answered, smiling.

"Once, a man came in carrying his own severed arm. I don't get shocked anymore."

In the UK, North America and other parts of the world, medical specialties and subspecialties abound, and more are created as our knowledge grows. Many doctors are becoming super-specialists, knowing more and more about less and less, while generalists are a dying breed. As a barrister, I often use medical experts who specialise in the shoulder, or the hand, or the knee. A general orthopaedic surgeon will no longer do.

In rural Tamil Nadu, surgeons, anaesthetists, paediatricians, and other specialists do general outpatient work, as well as their specialist cases. If stranded on a desert island with the choice of a single doctor, an Indian-trained rural surgeon would be a wise choice.

As my time in India neared its end, I reflected on the lessons learnt. The single greatest lesson was a reaffirmation of Jean Bernard's observation that medicine is fundamentally about man. The common feature transcending all of medicine is that each practitioner, whatever his specialty, location, or century, aims ultimately for the good of man, often at a time of vulnerability and weakness. This obvious truth, in this era of specialisation, technology, stringent rules and protocols, can quite easily be forgotten.

It is also a team effort. An operation, for example, is not a tête-à-tête between a surgeon and a patient. It may involve a small crowd of nurses, assistants, anaesthetists, surgeons, and students.

Man's involvement at both the giving and receiving

end of medicine makes it a fallible and challenging affair. When it works, however, even in the most remote corners of the world, the flickering star of humanity twinkles.

HOW TO TREAT A PIRAHÃ: MEDICAL ETHICS AND CULTURAL DIFFERENCE

Deep in the Amazon rainforest the Pirahã (pronounced pee-da-HAN) people speak a language unlike any other. The language has only 3 vowels and 8 consonants and has no numbers, no counting, and no words for colours. A Pirahã would refer to red, for example, by saying, "That is like blood."

The Pirahã have minimal art and no musical instruments. They have no interest in the distant past or future. They ascribe scant value to privacy and show little fear of death. They have no doctors or hospitals. Yet, even the Pirahã have principles of medical ethics. The linguistics expert Dan Everett, who spent many years among the Pirahã, tells of a group of men killing a very sick baby by pouring copious amounts of alcohol in its mouth. He explained: "They felt certain that this baby was going to die. They felt it was suffering terribly [...] So they euthanised the child." All cultures have moral rules about the practice of medicine.

Doctors in this country are unlikely ever to treat a Pirahã, but they will certainly encounter patients from cultures very different from their own. This can create legal and ethical difficulties. The prosecution in 2015 of a gynaecologist for restitching the labia of a circumcised woman after she gave birth serves as a cautionary tale. The prosecution alleged that the procedure was contrary to section 1 of the Female Genital Mutilation Act 2003. Section 1(1) of the act stipulates: "A person is guilty of an offence if he excises, infibulates or otherwise mutilates the whole or any part of a girl's labia majora, labia minora or clitoris." Although female genital cutting is common in dozens of countries in Africa and the Middle East (in Somalia and Guinea over 90% of women are cut), the doctor had never treated a circumcised woman, nor received any relevant training.

Respecting a patient's culture can conflict with an ethical or legal duty. Anglo-American medical ethics is individualistic. By contrast, traditional Chinese medical ethics and some strands of African bioethics focus on community or family autonomy rather than individual autonomy. A patient is considered part of a family, with a system of hierarchy and seniority. This may result in relatives asking doctors to withhold a grim diagnosis or prognosis from a patient, for example. Withholding such news may be culturally appropriate but can undermine the validity of a patient's consent to subsequent treatment: the consent would be based on incomplete information.

Clinicians in England should respect a patient's cultural preferences so long as this does not breach guidelines of the GMC, English law, or fundamental tenets of medical ethics. When in doubt, a prudent clinician will seek advice. Clinical colleagues and hospital chaplains are handy sources of advice, but all doctors would do well to keep on their phones the number of the BMA ethics hotline, the hospital's clinical ethics committee, or some equivalent resource.

As patients and relatives, we should explain the significance of any cultural practices that may be alien to the medical team but, at the same time, must refrain from asking clinicians to act unlawfully or contrary to their conscience or professional rules. They too have an autonomy that should be respected.

The importance of cultural competence in medicine is well recognised. The GMC, in *Good Medical Practice*, reminds doctors that "in assessing what is of overall benefit to adult patients" they must "take into account their cultural, religious, or other beliefs and values." This requires a flexibility of mind and openness that comes naturally to some and not to others.

The efforts to contain Ebola in West Africa during the 2013-2015 outbreak and the work of military medics abroad have highlighted the value of cultural sensitivity. In the Ebola epidemic, a key source of spread was the burials. They accounted for at least 20% of new Ebola infections. Local customs often involved the kissing, washing, and touching of the bodies with bare hands, and distributing personal belongings of the deceased to loved ones. Dr Pierre Formenty, an Ebola expert who worked for the World Health Organization, observed: "Introducing components such as inviting the family to be involved in digging the grave and offering options for dry ablution and shrouding will make a significant difference in curbing Ebola transmission."

Here is a military example. An Afghan boy picks up a bomb that explodes in his right hand, causing very severe injuries. Should the doctors amputate the hand? That decision is not solely medical. The clinicians must appreciate the cultural significance of losing a hand in that community. The left hand, which would be the boy's only remaining hand, is considered 'unclean'. Further, thieves are punished by amputation of the hand, and the boy might be mistakenly perceived as a thief. Without knowledge of the patient's culture, customs, and taboos, doctors risk making errors when balancing the harm and benefits of treatment options. The ethical principles of beneficence (doing good for the patient) and non-maleficence (not causing net harm) cannot be divorced from the broader social context.

At times, a clinician will need to suppress personal beliefs and prejudices. Part of being a doctor – and a lawyer, for that matter – entails keeping some of your thoughts to yourself and presenting a composed front to the patient. A disapproving attitude is unprofessional and can deter a patient, perhaps already embarrassed by their difference, from returning.

The plurality of cultures and traditions among patients can be baffling to those treating them and if ignored can lead to mistrust, poor care, and complaints. Beneath the surface, however, the core values of medicine remain unaltered. Medical morality emerges from a universal experience of a healer helping a fellow human being who is ill and suffering, be it a lord in London or a Pirahã in the Amazon. That most human of encounters between healer and patient transcends all cultures.

DOCTORS AND TORTURE IN IRAQ

It is a curious but well-known paradox that medicine has gained much from the horrors of war. Amputations, antisepsis, skin transplants, and the treatment of gunshot wounds were all greatly improved through observing and treating casualties of war. Wars naturally provide opportunities for doctors to perform heroic acts. Braving enemy fire, the French military surgeon Dominique Larrey (1766-1842) rode into the battlefield to treat and evacuate wounded soldiers, performing dozens of emergency amputations. In times of war, military doctors have fulfilled two obligations: to treat patients and to serve their country.

In the Iraq war that started in 2003, these two obligations came into conflict. During interrogations, military doctors were asked to participate in acts of torture and humiliation. The persons before them were both patients and enemies. According to the interrogation manual issued to the US military, doctors were required to supervise interrogation techniques, such as food deprivation, and to ensure that prisoners were fit for interrogation.

Aside from actively participating in torture, doctors

around the world have also been – and continue to be in countries such as North Korea, China, Uzbekistan, Syria, Guyana, and many others – complicit in torture by designing methods of torture that leave no scars, ensuring that victims do not die from their injuries, failing to report seeing patients who have been tortured, and failing to record signs and symptoms of torture in medical records or death certificates.

A recent article in the *BMJ* by researchers at the University of California, San Francisco, discussed the role of clinicians in the solitary confinement of prisoners in US prisons, referring to the case of Arthur Johnson. Until his court-ordered release into the general prison population in September 2016, Johnson had been in solitary confinement, in a small cell with lights kept on for prolonged periods, for a staggering 36 years. The authors concluded that his healthcare providers "gave a clinical endorsement of Johnson's mental fitness for indefinite isolation, violating ethical proscriptions against participation in punishment, particularly forms amounting to torture."

One Iraqi woman, who was tortured in Abu Ghraib prison, told Amnesty International that prisoners were often unconscious after interrogation sessions. Two doctors, usually one American and one Iraqi, then examined the prisoners. On one occasion, a doctor was ordered to insert an intravenous catheter into the corpse of a prisoner killed under interrogation to disguise the cause and time of death. Military doctors thus faced a conflict between their ethical duties to patients and their obligation to obey the orders of those higher in command.

The primary aim – or *telos* – of medicine is the alleviation of suffering. The Hippocratic oath, written in the 5th century BC, is clear on this: "I will use my power to help the sick to the best of my ability and judgment; I will abstain from harming or wronging any man by it". The consequent prohibition of torture is echoed by many contemporary codes of ethics, such as the World Medical Association's Declaration of Tokyo, the United Nations Convention against Torture, and the European Convention on Human Rights.

Medical doctors, both civilian and military, have a dual obligation to benefit their patients and to avoid causing them harm. Involvement in torture, even passively, infringes both these obligations. No other activity so violates the fundamental tenets of the medical profession. In such situations, the line separating doctors from torturers is blurred. There is little moral difference between starving a prisoner by withholding food and *supervising* the starvation of a prisoner, or between electrocuting a prisoner and ensuring that the prisoner can be 'safely' electrocuted.

Only a credible threat to one's own life, or the life of loved ones, may arguably justify participating in torture. This was the case for some Iraqi doctors under Saddam Hussein, who were forced to participate under threat of death to themselves and their families by Uday Hussein's (Saddam's eldest son) paramilitary forces. Western military doctors, however, were not acting under duress. Dr Steven Miles, an ethicist and expert in the role of doctors in torture, said in an interview for *The Atlantic* that doctors who "get involved in this [torture], number one, are careerists. They get involved for rank and career, and the regimes never coerce them, or extremely rarely coerce them. Instead what happens is the regimes treat them as some kind of elite."

The oath refers not only to doctors' ability, but also their judgment. Both these skills are required for the safe and ethical practice of medicine. While doctors who possess only technical ability are a threat to their patients, so too are doctors of sound judgment but inadequate knowledge. It is judgment that the military doctors in Iraq most needed when faced with their conflict of duties. How should they have balanced the duty of care to their patients with the duty to fulfil military objectives?

In a speech to newly trained army surgeons in 1894, Sir William Osler issued some precautionary advice to his audience: "do not forget that, though army officers, you owe allegiance to an honourable profession, to the members of which you are linked by ties of a most binding character". For Osler, the ethical scales with patients on one side and country on the other tipped to the side of the patients.

Deliberately mistreating patients, for whatever seemingly noble reason, is contrary to the telos of medicine. The bond between doctor and patient is tighter than the impersonal, abstract relationship between a doctor and the military objectives of those in command.

The objectives of a doctor caring for a patient will always be laudable. No hindsight will ever cast scorn or criticism on a doctor's efforts to reduce suffering, but the objectives of military commanders or political leaders may be, and historically often have been, misguided.

THE MEDICAL ETHICS OF THE BATTLEFIELD

Athena, goddess of war, gave Asclepius two vials of the Medusa's blood. The blood from the Medusa's left side could raise the dead; the blood from the right side could kill instantly. The descendants of Asclepius – the thousands of medics who today grace the battlefields of the world – rarely use the right-sided blood. Battlefield euthanasia, in which death is hastened to avoid prolonged suffering, is a controversial practice, but it is as old as war itself and, whatever laws or rules prohibit it, will doubtless continue until wars cease.

When reflecting on battlefield euthanasia, one story springs to mind, recounted to me by a clinical ethicist when I was an intern in clinical ethics in Mount Sinai Hospital in Toronto.

In June 2002, an elderly patient in the intensive care unit of a big hospital asked to see the clinical ethicist. Eleanor Jones, 82, was suffering from advanced liver cancer. Her doctors did not expect her to survive into the next month. To the ethicist's surprise, it was neither the cancer nor the fear of death that troubled her, but an event that took place over half a century before.

In January 1942, Eleanor Jones was posted as a military nurse in a hospital in Penang, Malaysia.

Despite numerous attempts by the British to hold off their advances, the Imperial Japanese Army were rapidly advancing on their position. In light of the imminent threat, Nurse Eleanor and the rest of the hospital residents were ordered to evacuate the area. All ambulatory patients and staff were to walk 11 miles over difficult terrain to be picked up by British naval ships. They would then be evacuated to Singapore for safety. As this was a military hospital, there were 126 soldiers who were either too ill or too injured to walk the distance. They had no choice but to remain in the hospital.

At the time, the usual practice for the Japanese army was to kill the bed-ridden soldiers with bayonets, and either kill or imprison the rest. Aware of their fate, some patients asked the doctors and nurses to leave them lethal doses of medication so that they could commit suicide before the arrival of the enemy. Others, too burned or wounded even to move, asked Nurse Eleanor to place the medication directly in their mouths. Some patients, soldiers to the end, requested hand grenades to "at least kill a few of the enemy" as they entered the hospital.

The medical team were faced with a range of moral dilemmas. Should they accede to the patients' requests? Should they leave the medication by their patients' bedside tables? Should they actively administer the lethal doses of medication to those too infirm to commit suicide? Should they provide the hand grenades to those eager to die in battle? And, most of all, should they escape with all the others or stay behind to care for their patients? Many people in the medical team felt unable to abandon their patients, irrespective of their patients' fate. However grim the prognosis, they believed that their duty to care transcended all personal risk and remained until their patients' expiring breath. Even the possibility of death and the certainty of their capture did not deter them from their duty to care.

In the end, encouraged by the doomed patients to flee and save their own lives, Nurse Eleanor and most of the hospital staff escaped. Yet, despite the patients' orders, the doctors and nurses drew lots to decide who would remain with them. Although each was given the possibility to opt out, no one refused to participate in the lottery. Two nurses stayed behind.

As it turned out, neither Eleanor nor the rest escaped. The ships carrying the escapees did not reach the shores of Singapore, but were sunk by Japanese war planes. Eleanor and many others were taken prisoner, while others were either shot or drowned. Sixty years later, days before her death, Eleanor Jones still wondered whether she had made the right decisions that day in January 1942.

The ethicist's advice was brief: "You are not to blame and have nothing to regret."

In the rest of this chapter, I wish to focus on the dilemmas associated with the blood from the left side of the Medusa. When should it be used and when foregone? And who should benefit from it?

The ability to maintain the wounded alive is nothing less than astounding. Medical advances combined with improved body armour and rapid evacuation have resulted in lives saved that would have been unsalvageable only 20 years ago.

As a member of the UK's Ministry of Defence's Research Ethics Committee, I was invited to Headley Court, the Defence Medical Rehabilitation Centre. The visit brought home the remarkable recoveries of soldiers who, weeks before, were lying on the battlefield on the brink of death. However, as in the civilian setting, the power to revive the dying has brought with it a host of ethical difficulties.

In one scenario, a member of the local security forces has suffered massive injuries from an improvised explosive device (IED). He has lost both his legs and both his forearms. The blast has removed his entire face. Tourniquets are controlling the bleeding from the legs. He is still alive. If he can be saved using the state-of-the-art medical services of the coalition, what of his future once transferred to a local health facility, whose facilities pale in comparison?

One Canadian paramedic working in Kandahar, Afghanistan, in 2007 described the transfer of patients to the local hospital as a "death sentence". The hospital had no ventilators, resuscitation equipment, laryngoscope, or monitoring devices. Dr Kevin Patterson, a Canadian doctor also posted in Afghanistan, recalls a mass casualty incident involving a mixture of coalition personnel and Afghans. The doctors were told not to intubate any of the Afghans with burns exceeding 50%. Without a burns unit, those patients would be doomed. The coalition patients, on the other hand, could be repatriated to their home countries and obtain high quality burn care. Such divergent treatment is hard to bear and highlights the need to develop local healthcare infrastructure, but what are the immediate alternatives?

Athena's vials are exhaustible, and resource issues can also plague the military medic. Beds, staff, and stocks are limited. Our patient might single-handedly drain the hospital's blood bank, leaving nothing in reserve for future casualties. The 3rd revision of the US Department of Defence's manual *Emergency War Surgery* states that "the decision to commit scarce resources cannot be based on the current tactical/medical/logistical situation alone". Such decisions should be made with an eye to the future.

If our Afghan patient is treated and survives to discharge, what kind of life awaits him back in his Afghan village, where the realities of survival and attitudes to profound disability may be a far cry from our own? This question cannot be answered without an understanding of the local culture, religion, and outlook. It is morally dangerous to uniformly impose our interpretation of when it is desirable to live or die, dismissing the patient's views as backward, barbaric, or misguided.

If the decision to treat is made, the patient will need to be evacuated. A Medical Emergency Response Team (MERT) helicopter can arrive within minutes to provide advance life support and whisk our patient off to intensive care at a 'role 3' medical facility. However, there is another consideration. Every excursion by the MERT carries risk. The helicopter is vulnerable and prone to enemy ground fire, and this additional danger must be factored into the decision.

There is another factor, relevant in this context but seldom encountered in civilian medical ethics: morale. General Dwight Eisenhower called morale the "greatest single factor in successful wars". Allowing the soldier to die on the battlefield can damage the morale of the troops. It smacks of abandonment. The fact that the patient is Afghan provides an added reason to evacuate him, for not doing so may cause other Afghans to lose faith in the commitment of their fighting partners.

In October 2010, the Defence Medical Services (DMS) organised a day-long meeting to discuss some of the ethical issues facing medical personnel in the field, including scenarios such as the ones in this chapter. It was a significant step, a recognition that pre-deployment training should include an appreciation of the ethical challenges that can otherwise startle the unwary medic. When Athena gave Asclepius the vials, she did not provide advice on their use. The DMS sought to fill that gap. I cannot remember the last time I left a conference with so many unanswered questions swirling in my mind.

After the meeting, I was involved in the development of the Ministry of Defence's *Medical Ethics Guidelines for Operations*, which provided practical guidance for military doctors deployed in war zones.

The International Committee of Military Medicine

now organises an annual workshop in military medical ethics, and the literature on the subject, though still relatively small, is growing. My hope is that experts from relevant fields will devote more attention to one of the most challenging, important, and fascinating areas of medical ethics.

THE ESSENCE OF MEDICINE

AN ETHICIST IN THE NEUROLOGY DEPARTMENT

When I was working as a lecturer in medical ethics over a decade ago, a neurologist asked if I wanted to see a patient with the medical students. I accepted.

I don't know whether the patient expected this: a crowd of 10 curious students in this small, overlit room deep in the bowels of the hospital. She seemed so exposed and frightened in her wheelchair, like a hapless musician unwittingly pushed on stage. The neurologist, standing by her side, was hitting a tendon hammer against his palm.

"Please gather around," he ordered, "and get as close as you can to the patient." We encircled her. A student in the front row took a history.

Anastasia Hayes (who wishes to have her name published) was in her 60s, with golden hair and thick glasses that magnified her eyes. Her voice was soft, close to a whisper. She explained how, months ago, her left leg had become weak. Then the weakness had spread to her right hand. "I thought it was just one of those things," she said. Today Anastasia cannot get changed or wash herself unassisted. When the neurologist asked her to walk from one end of the room to the other, she dragged her foot along the floor, as if lugging a rock-filled sack. Walking was a Sisyphean struggle, each laboured step making way for the next.

She was asked to lie on the bed. "I don't think I can," she murmured, with a hint of embarrassment. Two students helped her onto the bed. One by one the students performed various tests. They pushed and pulled and hit and scratched, some with confidence, others with timidity. As the crowd admired a performance of Babinski's reflex, I saw Anastasia glance at her watch. It was lonely at her end. An hour had passed.

"I had never heard of motor neurone disease," she said after the physical examination, sitting once again in her wheelchair. "They gave me some leaflets, but I couldn't bring myself to read them."

"What did the doctor tell you about the disease?" the neurologist asked, crouching next to her. The room was silent.

"He said I'm going to have trouble moving my arms and legs. That I'll have trouble breathing… and swallowing." Anastasia spoke hesitantly, as if remembering a half learnt poem. Then she paused, and the silence became louder. "It's going to be tough."

Behind her glasses, tears welled up in her eyes. She wiped them away and apologised.

Overwhelmed with sadness, I felt like a voyeur, peering through her glasses into the recesses of her stricken soul. I did not understand why she apologised. What rule did she transgress? The rule of optimism? Of stoicism? Of dry eyed composure?

At first, I blamed the neurologist for her distress. Why did he ask the dreaded question? He, of all people, must have known the grim future awaiting her. The medical students, in their penultimate year, knew. Even I knew. I also blamed him for my own discomfort.

This was not part of the deal when he invited me to attend his class. This was too close and too real for an academic ethicist. We need distance, physical and emotional, to think objectively on ponderous matters. Detachment is essential to clear thinking.

Earlier that day, on the bus to work, I had reread an essay by Richard Selzer, a master of both pen and scalpel, in search of advice for a surgeon friend. The day before, my friend had confessed: "I just had to break terrible news to a patient. His tumour is inoperable. But I didn't feel sad at all. I was unmoved."

On the bus, I eventually found the passage I had in mind. It starts thus: "A surgeon does not slip from his mother's womb with compassion smeared upon him like the drippings of his birth. It is much later that it comes."

Selzer writes that a surgeon's compassion arises from the "cumulative murmuring of the numberless wounds he has dressed, the incisions he has made, all the sores and ulcers and cavities he has touched in order to heal." I emailed the extract to my friend, hoping that he might draw some comfort from it, and went about my day.

Drying the last of her tears, Anastasia said, "I hope I'll be strong enough to cope." The neurologist squeezed her hand. He did not say a word. As I watched him comfort the patient, my thoughts returned to Selzer's essay and his concluding words: "Out of the resonance between the sick man and the one who tends him there may spring that profound courtesy that the religious call Love."

As I read the essay on the bus, it occurred to me that Paracelsus in the 16th century and the late French haematologist Jean Bernard also claimed that medicine was grounded on love. There must be some truth in this, I told myself, as the bus arrived at my stop, but the idea remained hazy in my mind, a little too poetic.

In that silent moment of compassion when the neurologist squeezed Anastasia's hand, even in the presence of 10 medical students, I caught a glimpse of it. It was more subtle even than the patient's barely visible fasciculation. The words of Paracelsus, Bernard, and Selzer, which hours earlier had sounded fuzzy, now rang out with a newfound clarity. I saw, for the first time, the very essence of medicine.

WONDER IN MEDICINE

The lectures we attend, like the articles we read, seldom withstand the ravages of memory. Two lectures, however, are etched in my mind. The first was delivered to all of 3 students by a professor of romance languages. Its unpromising topic was morphology (which in linguistics concerns the structure of words). The second, by a member of the Inner Magic Circle of London, was on showmanship. He revealed the secrets of turning ordinary tricks into full-blown miracles. More than mastery of their subject, the two lecturers had the panache of Cyrano. They also exuded a profound sense of wonder – a wonder at the magic of language and the beauty of a visual illusion.

The Greeks called this sense of wonder or bewilderment 'thauma'. Plato believed it "the mark of the philosopher", and his student Aristotle considered it the precursor to wisdom, for it forms the starting point of philosophy. Leafing through the patients' notes of the neurosurgeon Harvey Cushing, I found this sense of wonder to leap out from his writings, photographs, and hand-drawn sketches. He viewed the pituitary gland and its disorders with awe. Another US surgeon, Sherwin Nuland, admits in his book on the history of human organs that his "fascination with medicine has been renewed over and over again by challenging and exhilarating contacts with patients, disease, and the response of the organs of the body."

Clinicians, medical ethicists and lawyers are regularly confronted with odd or extraordinary situations, and there is something amiss if even as experienced professionals we are no longer astonished by these situations. Such indifference may indicate a lack of humility, for to experience wonder we must be attuned to our limits and ignorance. So vast is the field of medicine that the most accomplished doctor will be familiar with little more than a speck. To paraphrase Cushing, the kaleidoscope of medicine is constantly turning. No individual can singlehandedly master the subject.

Much of our work, it is true, is not wonder-full. Filling forms, dictating letters in the clinic, or marking hundreds of exam scripts is underwhelming. Even in the humdrum, however, glimpses can be caught. Reading a student's essay, I was looking for a tree and a sturdy piece of rope when I stumbled on this sentence: "All humans should be treated with equal prejudice." Once my laughter had subsided, the phrase triggered a stream of thought about my own biases and prejudices (prejudiced, moi?) and about whether it was possible or even desirable to identify and remove them all.

In writing this chapter, I asked medical friends and colleagues about their work. A pathologist at the autopsy table, cupping a brain in his hands, describes

74

his unwavering fascination with the human body: "I've been cutting bodies for years, and I'm still baffled by it all." He places the patient's organs in a plastic bag, dumps the bag in the eviscerated chest, and sews it shut. Across the room, clearing the table of clotted blood, his colleague tells me of the beauty she finds in looking at microscopic images of defective tissue. The Czech immunologist Miroslav Holub called these cellular vistas "dreaming landscapes". All the while, the corpse's eyes remain open. I try to avoid her gaze.

Watching yet another appendix ensnared laparoscopically I ask the general surgeon if he ever tires of appendicectomies. I was bored after seeing a dozen. "Oh no!" he replied. "They're all different." I ask a GP colleague whether she still experiences wonder in her work, after nearly 20 years of practice. She recounts a recent house visit to an elderly couple who had devoted their lives to caring for their disabled adult children. She said: "I thought, 'Wow! These parents are doing a superhuman job!' That sort of case is quite unusual, but even in my everyday work I'm surprised by how people cope with a lot of shit, frankly."

Of all the professions, few contain as much potential for bafflement as medicine. The varied manifestations and effects of disease – be it an ossifying fibroma as large as a watermelon, or the vascular devastation of a haemorrhagic fever, the fortitude of a patient faced with impending death, or the devotion of carers to fellow human beings – can each trigger a sense of wonder.

We also wonder at the skill and wisdom of colleagues,

whether in person or through their writings. We recall our admiration when seeing the masterly actions of a mentor: the calm composure in a moment of crisis, the brilliant diagnosis that stumped colleagues, the comforting word or look that soothed a patient's pain. And, as Ralph Waldo Emerson noted in his essay *The Poet*, words are also actions. It would have taken me years, if not a lifetime, to acquire the insights on end of life care that Dr Joseph Fins, physician and Professor of Medical Ethics, shared in his 2005 book *A Palliative Ethic of Care*.

In our hectic, time-starved schedule, it can be difficult to pause and ponder on the wonder inherent in our work. But it is there, and it is worth noting, lest we allow the twin threats of apathy and arrogance to calcify in our cranium.

FIRST DO NOT HARM REVISITED

Clinicians of every ilk enjoy aphorisms. Favourites include "time is brain" (if a patient suffers a stroke, the longer you leave it, the more likely brain tissue will be damaged) and "common things are common".

Yet, surely no medical saying is better known than "first do no harm" or, to use the Latin phrase, "primum non nocere". PubMed shows that there are currently 358 articles with "first do no harm" in the title. Amazon shows 108 books with those words in the title.

Contrary to popular belief the phrase does not appear in the Hippocratic oath or the Hippocratic corpus (Hippocrates wrote in Greek, not Latin). Rather, the saying is attributed to Thomas Inman, as recently as 1860. That same year Oliver Wendell Holmes Senior famously remarked in a lecture to the Massachusetts Medical Society, "If the whole material medica [the drugs and remedial products], as now used, could be sunk to the bottom of the sea, it would be all the better for mankind – and all the worse for the fishes." He observed that the injuries caused by overmedication were often masked by the disease.

"First do no harm" remains an important injunction against overtreatment.

A few years ago, I was sitting on a hospital ethics committee reviewing the case of a woman who had just died from cancer. After the chairman read out the interminable list of treatments and procedures she had undergone, a consultant commented, "Wow, it's difficult to die in this hospital!"

Like many axioms or aphorisms, "first do no harm" is a crude piece of advice. Clinicians inflict harm all the time, whether it is by inserting a cannula, administering chemotherapy, performing a tracheotomy, opening an abdomen, or drilling into the skull. Most attempts to benefit a patient require the infliction of harm or, at the very least, involve risks of harm. The clinician's hope is that the benefits will outweigh the harm. A literal reading of "first do no harm" would, therefore, lead the clinician to do nothing at all.

A more accurate formulation is "first do no *net* harm". The Latin translation does not roll off the tongue: "primum non plus nocere quam succurrere" ("above all, do not harm more than succour").

At an individual level, clinicians must balance their obligation to benefit the patient (the principle of beneficence) against their obligation not to cause harm (the principle of non-maleficence). These twin obligations go hand in hand and are weighed against each other.

At times, it is difficult to evaluate which trumps the other, as the risks and benefits are unclear. There is considerable debate, for example, on the appropriateness of decompressive craniectomy after severe traumatic brain injury. The procedure involves removing part of the skull to allow the injured brain to swell to reduce intracranial pressure. The operation may lower the chance of death but can leave survivors with profound disabilities.

The decision will be informed by the clinical facts, but the harm-benefit analysis will also involve value judgments about what constitutes an acceptable risk or an acceptable quality of life. The same applies, for example, in decisions on whether to perform a tracheotomy on a critically ill patient. If a terminally ill patient might survive an additional six months with aggressive care, should the tracheotomy be done?

A wise clinician will say, "It depends partly on what the patient wants." The perception of what constitutes a harm and a benefit varies from person to person. In many situations the patient can tell the medical team how he or she balances the harm and benefits. Given this variability, the principles of beneficence and non-maleficence are best assessed in light of the principle of respect for autonomy. However, in cases of severe injury, including those where decompressive craniectomy is contemplated, patients may be unable to express their autonomous preferences. Well drafted advance directives can obviate such problems, but these documents are still rare in Britain.

The application of "first do no net harm" also arises at the interpersonal level. In vaccination programmes the balancing exercise is usually straightforward. The benefits to the many will outweigh the harm to the few. In other contexts the exercise will be fraught with difficulty. In an article in the *Journal of Clinical Ethics* a doctor recalled a dilemma she faced when working in a hospital in Port-au-Prince, Haiti, after the 2010 earthquake. Four patients presented in respiratory distress. There were no ventilators and only one oxygen tank.

One patient was a neurologically devastated 15-year-old girl with treatable pneumonia. Another was a 40-year-old woman with HIV, suspected tuberculosis, and three young children at her bedside imploring the staff for help. Another was a 25-year-old nurse with a probable pulmonary embolism resulting from major bowel surgery. The fourth patient was a beautiful 18-year-old girl with acute decompensated heart failure.

The doctor's first choice was the nurse, even though the 15-year-old was the most medically salvageable in the short term. The doctor asked, "Did I make a medical judgment based on a co-morbidity, or a value judgment based on my own latent biases? I am honestly not sure." This dilemma shows that balancing harm and benefits is not a purely clinical exercise.

On close inspection "first do no harm" is a flawed dictum. "First do no net harm" is better but still needs to be interpreted in the context of other moral principles, such as justice and respect for autonomy.

MATTERS OF LIFE AND DEATH AND
QUALITY OF LIFE

Some doctors deal with matters of life and death on a
regular basis. If the cardiac surgeon ignores the leaking
aneurysm, the patient will die in minutes. If the
anaesthetist fails to intubate at once, the patient will
asphyxiate. In an emergency department in the United
States I was present when a patient shot through the back
was admitted by helicopter, his chest opened up within
seconds of landing, and his heart pumped manually
by a trauma physician. It was impressive, high octane
medicine.

In the course of a recent conversation with one of
those life and death doctors, I lamented the plight of a
young woman who had lost a leg in a road crash. Her
life had been forever changed. She could no longer do
things that we take for granted, such as swimming or
taking the train or wearing certain clothes. The doctor
remarked, to my surprise, that, though regrettable, "it
wasn't a matter of life and death."

This dismissive attitude reminded me of the
businessman character in Saint Exupéry's *Little Prince*. In
this novella the narrator is stranded in the desert when he
encounters a wise, otherwordly little prince who recounts

stories from his and other planets. The businessman inhabits one tiny planet. He spends his days counting stars for no apparent reason and repeatedly tells the little prince not to disturb him as he is concerned about "matters of consequence". The little prince's beloved single rose, unique and under threat on his planet, was in contrast inconsequential, the businessman says. There is no denying that it is important for a doctor to fix a damaged heart, and in some cases so too is counting stars, but the truth is that all doctors deal with matters of consequence. Hospital doctors hold no monopoly over such issues.

In one of John Mortimer's *Rumpole* stories, Rumpole, under strict instructions from his tyrannical wife, visits his general practitioner, Dr MacClintock, a "small, lightweight, puritanical Scot who looked as though he existed on a glass of cold water and a handful of Quaker Oats a day." At the end of the consultation Dr MacClintock tells his overweight patient, "Let's face the fact, there is a great deal too much of you, Mr Rumpole," and prescribes a Spartan diet of *Thin-O-Vite*. Life and death doctors might well concede that Dr MacClintock was dealing with a matter of life and death, albeit at a dull, chronic level. Without a change of diet, the fried slices, rashers of bacon, sausages, buttered crumpets, jam roly-poly, Château Thames Embankment, and small cigars so enjoyed by Rumpole would doubtlessly lead to an early demise.

But what of doctors who, instead of pumping the exposed hearts of mortally wounded patients, deal on a daily basis with blocked ears, sprained ankles, and other mundane afflictions?

When I was a law student I spent one evening a week at a community law centre, armed only with a meagre knowledge of the law and a dose of common sense, trying to solve the legal problems of the local folk: a tenant was tormented by voracious bed bugs, a young lady had lost her part time job for swearing at a customer, an impecunious student had squandered his savings on a broken computer on eBay, and other sorry tales of this sort. These were the law's equivalent of blocked ears and sprained ankles. Damages seldom exceeded a few hundred pounds. Yet, for the individuals involved, many of whom felt nervous just seeking legal help, these ostensibly trivial matters meant a great deal.

The same is true of patients. Whatever the doctor may think about their gravity, few of us visit the doctor for ailments we consider trivial. Like the little prince's rose, the problem is, to our eyes, important. A sound grasp of this fact lies at the heart of a good bedside manner. Excising a tumour may be more dramatic than removing wax from a person's ear or treating a corneal ulcer, but they are all potentially matters of consequence, looming large in the patient's consciousness. Each intervention shares the fundamental aim of improving quality of life. How I remember the awful days spent at home, afflicted by a corneal ulcer, half blind and in agony at every blink; and how blissful the relief when the drops prescribed by the ophthalmologist finally took effect.

In John Mortimer's story Dr MacClintock paradoxically drops dead in front of the bon vivant Rumpole, who, a glass of champagne in hand, muses, "It's the quality of life that matters, isn't it? The quality of life. And the hell with *Thin-O-Vite.*" What can be more important, more consequential, than the quality of one's life? Not all medical practice is a matter of life and death, but all medicine deals ultimately with quality of life.

In medical heaven I doubt that Hippocrates, Maimonides, Osler, or whoever it is who assesses the new entrants will look on the cardiac surgeon more favourably than the rural GP, or the ophthalmologist, on the basis of a crude life and death criterion.

MEDICINE'S SOLEMN MOMENTS

Not so long ago, at the start of a trial I took part in, the opposing barrister was ruffling through his papers while my witness was swearing the oath: "I swear by almighty God that I will tell the truth [ruffling of papers]... the whole truth [more ruffling]..." At this point the judge, with a frown, told my opponent to stop at once.

I was surprised by this judicial rebuke. Many barristers, for whom the court procedure has become second nature, pay little attention during the swearing of the oath. They arrange their papers, or re-read key documents, or fill a glass of water.

Yet the judge was right. Swearing an oath is a solemn moment, and the lawyers in the courtroom should behave accordingly. Now, during the oath, I keep as still as a statue and look the witness in the eye.

The death of the surgeon and writer Richard Selzer on 15th June 2016 prompted me to re-read some of his work. For those readers unfamiliar with his work, you should start with Mortal Lessons: Notes on the Art of Surgery and Letters to a Young Doctor.

I came across an interview Selzer gave to the writer Peter Josyph: "I was the commencement speaker at Boston University a couple of years ago. As we stood to recite the oath, I looked at the graduates, and I saw a couple of them laughing and snickering during the administration of the oath. I was offended down to my toes by that. I couldn't believe that anyone would be embarking upon this work and not be focused on the words of it."

In a blog on the Journal of Medical Ethics website, written on 23rd October 2017, Dr Iain Brassington, a Senior Lecturer in Bioethics at the University of Manchester, criticised the latest revision of the World Medical Association's Declaration of Geneva. The declaration, which sets out the ethical duties of doctors, is described on the WMA's website as the contemporary successor to the 2,500-year-old Hippocratic oath. The declaration starts: "As a member of the medical profession: I solemnly pledge to dedicate my life to the service of humanity." Brassington asks rhetorically, "What's the difference between a pledge and a solemn pledge?" Commenting on "I will foster the honour and noble traditions of the medical profession," he writes: "Huh? It's just a job, mate. Get over it."

Being a doctor is not 'just a job', or at least it should not be. It possesses a moral dimension not found in nearly all other jobs. Hence why there is no Professor in Baking Ethics, or Painting and Decorating Ethics, or Hairdressing Ethics, and why Selzer was so incensed when he saw the medical graduates making light of the oath. In the Hippocratic oath, the doctors swore by "Apollo, Asclepius, Hygieia, Panacea and by all the gods and goddesses". In the secular, modern-day version, doctors "solemnly" pledge. The purpose? To acknowledge the privilege, importance and dignity of treating a fellow human being in need.

There are events, such as the reciting of an oath, whose significance we may not fully appreciate until it is pointed out to us. The significance is lost through familiarity or lack of reflection.

More subtle examples of solemn moments exist in medicine. One is the signing of the consent form, an act so common that many doctors scarcely give it a thought. For the patient, however, it may be as rare as signing the register in a marriage ceremony. It is an expression of trust like no other.

When asking the patient to sign the consent form, the person seeking the consent should act in a way that reflects the significance of the act. In the moments between the invitation to sign and the signing itself there should be no joking, no talking, no fiddling with phones or bleeps. The doctor's demeanour will signify to the patient that this is an important occasion in the sacred relationship between doctor and patient.

Undoubtedly there are other solemn moments in the course of interactions with patients in rounds or clinics that, through habit, gradually lose their significance to become quite ordinary. It may be the giving of a diagnosis or prognosis or a physical examination.

One of Selzer's great contributions to medicine is showing us that these moments are more prevalent than we think.

EDUCATING DOCTORS

THE MESSINESS OF MEDICINE

A few years ago I attended a conference for surgeons. In the hall, a poster described the case of a neurology patient who had, literally, inhaled a chicken sandwich. The surgeon, with great ingenuity, combined instruments to suction the mushy chicken embedded in the patient's lungs.

Next to the poster stood a timid medical student, one of three authors on the poster, no doubt petrified at the prospect of senior doctors asking him about the minutiae of the novel procedure.

During a break, I encouraged the student – a bright and charming third year – to publish the poster as a case report. Suitably mollified, I asked him about his views on medical ethics. "I'm scientifically minded so I struggle with the fact that there's no clear answer in ethics," he replied.

And so I launched into some of my law cases. A doctor wrongly injected an anaesthetic into my client's spinal cord and left them with incomplete tetraplegia. The neurology experts, both holders of PhDs, could not agree on whether my client would develop multiple sclerosis. Neither could they agree by how many years the medical accident had reduced their life expectancy.

In another case, the patient collapsed at home the day after an operation and needed a corrective operation. One neurosurgeon felt that the patient should not have been discharged on the day of the operation, while another saw nothing wrong with that practice.

In yet another, an obstetrician believed suturing the internal anal sphincter after a deep tear following birth made all the difference, while a colorectal surgeon believed it did nothing at all.

In most cases that reach me, experienced consultants – experts in their discipline – disagree with each other on some fundamental aspect of clinical medicine, whether it's diagnosis, treatment, prognosis, or the general management of the patient.

Medical schools, perhaps for good reason, sanitise medicine to create the illusion that there are 'clean' answers: "Circle the correct answer on the multiple choice question." They downplay the uncertainty inherent in much of medical practice. Reading a scan, deciding to coil or clip an aneurysm, or even referring a patient to a specialist are, to some extent, matters of interpretation. Competent clinicians may come to different conclusions.

The idea for this chapter arose when, my monologue over, I saw the medical student's expression. He looked as if he had inhaled a chicken sandwich: "I never thought of it that way," he said. That observation, almost trite to medical lawyers and ethicists, was to him a revelation.

For lecturers faced with such 'scientifically minded'

students, pointing out the occasional messiness of medicine may make students more accepting of the occasional messiness of medical ethics.

As patients and relatives too, we should accept that medicine often cannot give the clear answer we so eagerly seek, whether the question is whether to undergo a major operation or whether our child has a viral or bacterial infection. Clinical uncertainty is common. If in doubt, ask your GP.

THE SIBERIAN TIGER

Cast your eye down the list of delegates at any course in medical ethics. You will find represented a wide range of specialties: the usual batch of GPs and anaesthetists, intensivists, psychiatrists, oncologists, junior doctors, and even the occasional radiologist and pathologist. Yet there is one species of doctor that is as rare as the Siberian tiger: the surgeon. I must confess that my eyes light up when I see a surgeon on the list, and I scan the room hoping to catch a glimpse of the rare animal.

When I see one in the flesh, he (for it usually is) tends, surprisingly, to be shy, crouching towards the back of the classroom or lecture theatre. More often than not he is an older creature. Without his tools and instruments, without his mask, exposed and alone, the surgeon on the ethics course has ventured into a foreign habitat.

The Royal College of Surgeons offers an extensive menu of training courses, from the cheerful drawing for surgeons to the bone-chilling course on the Ilizarov method. Although a course exists on legal issues in surgery, there is no course on surgical ethics. Several Royal Colleges, including those of the general practitioners, pathologists, obstetrics and gynaecology, paediatrics, and psychiatry, have established their own ethics committees. There is no such permanent committee for the surgeons.

Some of the surgical textbooks I consult on the library shelf have a few pages devoted to the law of consent, but ethics is notable by its absence. At surgical conferences oral presentations on the subject are rare. I was mightily surprised when, scanning the programme of the 14th European Congress on Neurosurgery, the last of the 42 topics was 'ethics in neurosurgery'. In my excitement I submitted an abstract in support of the brave surgeon who must have raised the idea to puzzled looks at a meeting of the scientific committee. As I was doing so, my wife, then a neurosurgical trainee, commented that this particular session would not be overflowing with delegates. No matter. A soliloquy is better than silence.

Surgery is a field brimming with ethical issues: a patient refuses lifesaving surgery on religious grounds or is the victim of an intraoperative error; another has been harmed by a previous doctor but knows nothing of it or has a tumour that is operable but high risk; and yet another mistakenly believes that the operator will be a consultant. There is also the sometimes tenuous link between properly informed consent and that signature on the consent form.

Incise deeper and you will find the surgeon who wants to try a new technique, the surgeon who adds his or her name to publications for no other reason than hierarchy, who is 'economical with the truth' with patients and family, whose hand is unsteady or whose judgment is impaired, whose tendency is to overtreat patients, or whose bedside manner borders on the discourteous. And what of the well intentioned but brash trainee who is unaware of his or her limits, the ethics regulating the proper relationship between the surgeon and the anaesthetist, or the ethics of operative scheduling and triaging, in ordinary times and in emergencies? And let us not forget the military surgeons, whose contributions to the art cannot be overestimated but whose ethical dilemmas are no less acute. The ethical issues are not visible on the radiologist's scan, nor palpable deep in the recesses of the iliac fossae, nor graspable like a bowel clamp, but are nevertheless there, as real and important as the potent gases of the anaesthetist.

Why there should be such a neglect of ethics training in surgery is unclear. I hope surgical readers will forgive me for suggesting the possibility of an irreverent attitude towards formal ethics education in surgery. Some of the older tigers may hold the attitude that junior surgeons learn ethics by copying their seniors and betters, that the ethics of surgery will enter the trainee like the absorbable sutures of the patient. Raanan Gillon, an Emeritus Professor of Medical Ethics (and author of the foreword to this book), encountered such a type when he expressed his desire to study for a PhD as a junior doctor in the 1960s. His consultant replied, in an incredulous tone, "You can't study medical ethics!" The main danger of the osmosis theory is that it can perpetuate bad habits, carefully developed over years of unethical conduct.

Another possibility, equally uncharitable, is that the decision makers in the surgical community, whose own training perhaps contained little ethics teaching, believe that there are few ethical issues in their specialty or that the issues are dealt with adequately in the Royal College of Surgeons' helpful booklet *Good Surgical Practice*. Alternatively they may think that these ethical issues are handled perfectly well at present and there is no need for change. "Seek and ye shall find" is the obvious response.

Talk to surgical trainees in private and, like their counterparts in medical specialties, they will soon complain about their need to publish articles and give presentations to further their careers. "What about something on ethics," I usually suggest, "perhaps an audit or a case report on an ethically interesting case?" Their response is that this would be received by their colleagues as enthusiastically as the wrong instrument in an operation. If my observations reflect the wider reality, the surgical community would benefit from a closer examination of the ethical issues in surgery. A one-day course in surgical ethics and law, the occasional session in conferences, the odd presentation at the weekly departmental meeting, and a word of encouragement at the mention of ethics. That is all. The rest will follow. Surgical ethics may not be very fashionable, but it is a central part of the practice of surgery.

In 100 years' time the Ilizarov method will be confined to the history books, but surgical ethics will endure.

AEQUANIMITAS

Few non-medical readers will have heard of Sir William Osler (1849-1919). Most doctors recognise the name because of Osler's nodes, small nodules on the fingers or toes which suggest a bacterial infection of the heart.

Osler was arguably the greatest doctor of all time. Born in Canada, he eventually became one of the founding Professors of Medicine at Johns Hopkins Hospital in Baltimore and, from 1905 to his death, Regius Professor of Medicine in Oxford. It is remarkable to think that, in 1892, Osler published what would become the most significant medical textbook of the early 20th century *single-handedly*. A similar textbook today would require hundreds of authors.

As well as his textbook, Osler wrote hundreds of educational and philosophical essays about the practice of medicine. I have long held the dangerous belief that Osler's essays, judiciously used, could render teachers of medical ethics redundant. Virtually all the medical student needs for ethical behaviour is contained within them.

One of Osler's most famous essays, *Aequanimitas*, was first delivered as a speech to newly minted doctors in 1889 at the Pennsylvania School of Medicine. Osler urges his young audience to "consider but two of the score of elements which may make or mar your lives." The first is imperturbability, which refers to "calmness amid storm, clearness of judgment in moments of grave peril."

This poker-faced composure, he claims, is essential to instil confidence in impressionable or frightened patients. Imperturbability is in part acquired through experience and a thorough knowledge of medicine. With these in hand, "no eventuality can disturb the mental equilibrium of the physician." We will return to imperturbability in the next chapter.

The second, related element – equanimity – has been the subject of some debate among Osler scholars. While some have interpreted it as apathy – the absence of emotions – others have read it as 'metriopatheia', measured or moderated emotions.

To acquire the virtue of equanimity, Osler recommends a tolerant, somewhat non-judgmental attitude towards our fellow humans. "The more closely we study their little foibles of one sort and another in the inner life which we see," he remarks, "the more surely is the conviction borne in upon us of the likeness of their weaknesses to our own." He continues: "The similarity would be intolerable, if a happy egotism did not often render us forgetful of it."

Osler also advises us not to seek certainty when it cannot be found but to be satisfied with fragments of the truth and to be ready for the inevitable struggles and disappointments ahead. When they arrive, "stand up bravely" and "wrestle on" with due persistence; and, should defeat come, cultivating a cheerful equanimity will make the pain easier to bear. When matters of principle or justice are in play, then "cling to your ideal", Osler urges, even in the face of evident failure. Osler's essay is a classic for several reasons.

Firstly, he tackles head-on a timeless question: what makes a good doctor? The ideals he proposes do not fade with passing years. His writing is meticulously crafted – each phrase, word, sound, and intonation deftly chosen, at times blurring the line between prose and poetry. Rich in cultural and literary allusions, the essay can be enjoyed by the teenage reader and erudite professor alike.

What is rare is that Osler's scholarship is not tainted by pretentiousness: "You remember in the Egyptian story, how Typhon with his conspirators dealt with good Osiris?" – well, no, I remember no such thing, but this ignorance engenders curiosity rather than shame. (Typhon and his conspirators did not deal kindly with his brother Osiris: they trapped him in a large chest, sealed it shut with molten lead, and threw it into the Nile.)

Even when discussing sombre matters Osler comes across as a benevolent presence, a calming hand on our shoulder: "It is sad to think, that for some of you, there is in store disappointment, perhaps failure."

My second-hand copy of *Aequanimitas* has written on the inside cover: "Presented by Charles E. Frosst & Co to G.E. Green on Graduation 1962". Charles

E. Frosst & Co was a pharmaceutical company, later acquired by Merck & Co. How infinitely more valuable a gift than the pens and selfie sticks that pharmaceutical companies now offer doctors at conferences!

HOW TO BE A COOL-HEADED CLINICIAN

At law school, as at medical school, however hard you study nothing quite prepares you for the real thing. In court, when your opponent rises to invoke an unfamiliar and potentially killer point, the mind tends to panic: "Where did this come from? Did I miss something in my preparation? What am I going to say?" Searching frantically for a response, you watch in despair as your opponent sits down. The stern looking judge nods expectantly in your direction: it is your turn to rise and speak. The world is now a lonely place, with nowhere to hide. Although stressful, this experience is central to professional development.

Experience alone, however, is of little value. The psychologist Anders Ericsson, an expert on experts, declared in a recent book that he had been "unable to find any evidence showing that experience has any benefits unless people pay attention to feedback and actively adjust." For it to be effective, experience must be reflected on.

I have got into the habit of jotting down key lessons after an eventful day in court. Recently, I simply wrote: "imperturbability".

Although empathy, compassion, and kindness are

buzz words in medical schools (so much so that some clinicians associate ethicists with bleeding hearts and sentimentality), William Osler told medical students in 1889, "In the physician or surgeon no quality takes rank with imperturbability. The physician who has the misfortune to be without it," Osler continued, "who betrays indecision and worry, and who shows that he is flustered and flurried in ordinary emergencies, loses rapidly the confidence of his patients." This appears at odds with the modern focus on empathy, but does Osler's view have a place in medical practice today?

It is often said that before the past few decades medical ethics emphasised manners, etiquette, and decorum, with empathy having only a small part to play. The importance of empathy today can be ascribed, at least in part, to the unprecedented use of technology in medicine; the limited time available to see patients; and the integration of communication skills, ethics, and the humanities in the medical curriculum. Empathy emerged as a counterpoint to the "stranger at the bedside" phenomenon, attempting to give the stranger a human face. The focus on empathy in the training of medical students has made the Oslerian virtue of imperturbability unfashionable.

A key problem with empathy is that it cannot readily be taught to those who are not, by nature, empathetic. You cannot teach empathy as you teach how to perform a lumbar puncture. In that respect, there is much to be said for focusing on less nebulous qualities, such as courtesy and politeness. These are undervalued traits in medicine, and although their importance may be obvious their application is more challenging in the heat of a busy clinic, when frustration and fatigue can test even the most patient doctor.

Aside from the difficulty in teaching empathy, it is debatable whether it is a desirable quality for doctors. Indeed, the ill effects of empathy underpin the reason why doctors should not treat loved ones. A degree of dispassion is needed to maintain a medical gaze not blurred by too great a concern for the patient as a person. Yet, the questionable benefits of empathy do not derogate from the importance of kindness, which is a less demanding emotion. Few patients would object to a kind doctor.

Many more would have concerns about an empathic doctor, fearing this shows either inexperience or a lack of mental fortitude. In the debates on the acceptability of doctors crying in front of patients, praying with them, or displaying outward effusions of emotion, at the risk of appearing heartless, I side with Osler. There must be an outward calm, a reassuring coolness, although it must not veer into indifference. Imperturbability is compatible with showing concern for the patient.

The million-dollar question is how to develop the quality of imperturbability, and here lessons can be gleaned from the world of elite performance. According to the Yale psychiatrist Andy Morgan, who has conducted research on stress in military trainees in the United States, perception is key: "How you frame something in your head has a great deal to do with your neurobiological response to it. Once you start saying to yourself, 'Oh my God, this is awful,' you begin releasing more cortisol and start this cascade of alarm."

Neuroscience is deepening our understanding of stress and decision-making, but it is clear that the poise of those doctors we admire is more than innate disposition. It requires repeated gritty experience and subsequent postmortems to discover what went right and wrong and to find ways to improve. This appreciation of the potential value of experience may, in itself, be reassuring next time an unexpected difficulty arises in the clinic, the operating theatre, or in Uxbridge County Court in front of a stone-hearted judge.

A PERFORATED EDUCATION

If asked to name famous doctors in medicine's long and tempestuous history, what would you say? Hippocrates, Galen, Avicenna, Maimonides, Vesalius, Harvey, Lister, Osler, Cushing, Salk?

When, as a Lecturer in Medical Ethics, I put this question to a class of third year medical students, I was disheartened to hear their first answer: Harold Shipman, the British GP who murdered more than 200 patients and hanged himself in prison in 2003. The next most popular answer was Gregory House, a brilliant though mischievous, cynical, and quite fictional character of the popular American television series *House*, starring Hugh Laurie.

A few years ago, I attended a surgical conference in London. A distinguished professor of surgery, who qualified in the first half of the 20th century, showed a chest X-ray to the audience. "We used to see a lot of this in the 1940s, when I was a house surgeon," he reminisced. With an austere nod of the head, he asked an unsuspecting junior doctor for a diagnosis. Junior doc: "I guess it could be..." Surgeon: "Don't guess, boy!" Junior doc (startled): "Is it a diaphragmatic hernia?" Surgeon: "I discard you like a perforated condom."

As I heard "Harold Shipman" and "*House*" leave the lips of those medical students, the surgeon's colourful dismissal seemed apposite.

It is perhaps unrealistic to expect students to know more than the basics of the profession's history, but surely every medical student worth their stethoscope should be familiar with the bare bones of the subject. Aside from history's intrinsic interest, it can foster a sense of perspective and continuity, and a spirit of reflective inquiry. Physician-historians have written about how knowledge of medical history has improved their clinical practice, from preventing hubris to aiding diagnosis.

Even a single session would benefit the student, and in answer to the obvious rejoinder, "If history creeps into the curriculum, what goes out?", I again suggest medical ethics, whose lessons can easily be incorporated into a history lecture. Medical history is replete with ethical issues.

So I spent the next 30 minutes of the class discussing key moments in medical history: the transition from a supernatural to a rational model of disease, Galen's humoral theory, vaccination, antisepsis, the germ theory of disease, and so on. For the last part of the hour, we dissected William Osler's essay *Teacher and Student*, in which Osler reflects on the characteristics of a good medical student and doctor.

He writes of the art of detachment, the virtue of method, the quality of thoroughness, and the grace of humility. I asked the students about the importance of these qualities. We discussed the meaning of humility and the benefits of the virtue: the ability to identify and learn from our mistakes, to learn from others, to gauge our abilities, and make more balanced judgments about others.

And inevitably, when the time came to discuss witnessed instances – or notable absences – of humility, the students invoked the cold hearted surgeon as the antithesis of humility. Where, in our hospitals, is the sensitive surgeon of TS Eliot's *East Coker*?

> *The wounded surgeon plies the steel*
> *That questions the distempered part;*
> *Beneath the bleeding hands we feel*
> *The sharp compassion of the healer's art*
> *Resolving the enigma of the fever chart.*

Jotted down on a Post-it note, a quote from the surgeon Richard Selzer dangles precariously on my computer: "The surgeon must remain anesthetized to the philosophical, the literary, even the human implications of his work, in order to be able to carry it out dispassionately, at the proper remove from the white heat of the event." How, if at all, can we reconcile these two extracts?

After the class, I bumped into one of the students on the underground. "How did you find the class?" I asked, aware that any positive answer would be borne out of politeness. "It was thought-provoking, but the guy next to me didn't see how it could help in exams." I discard you like…

Call me naive, but is there not something amiss about contemporary medical education when frequent examinations stifle the intellectual meanderings so essential for an expanded mind? In 1954, a 12-year-old boy in the United States wrote to Mr Justice Frankfurter, an eminent Supreme Court judge, requesting advice for a career in law. The judge recommended that the boy read widely for "no one can be a truly competent lawyer unless he is a cultivated man." Is that, I wonder, also true of medicine?

THE ETHICS CHECKLIST

It's the morning round in the hospital. In a dreary voice the doctor presents the patient, a 43-year-old man with fever, chills, and a productive cough. He has a new diagnosis of HIV infection. He is married and has a girlfriend. The two bioethicists in the room, hitherto lulled by the long list of treatments, stir uncomfortably in their seats: there may be problems afoot. Do the wife and girlfriend know about each other? Can the team distinguish one from the other? Does the patient want to share the diagnosis with either? Should they be told of their likely exposure to HIV, even without the patient's consent?

The purpose of oral presentations in rounds is to tell the patient's story. It is primarily a medical story, which may start before the patient's birth (if genetics are relevant) and extend to the future. The narrative helps the healthcare team make sense of the patient's situation and provide safe, effective care. Although the stories should be comprehensive, they are often incomplete. The ethical aspects are omitted.

At present the healthcare team has to tease these out from a heap of medical information. Sometimes the ethical issues stay buried in the heap, unnoticed. To reduce the risk of the clinical obscuring the ethical, a new section is needed in patients' notes.

The new category, named 'ethical issues', would consist of a short list of headings. It would not require much time to complete, nor would it require much knowledge of medical ethics. It would make explicit the key ethical issues of a case, helping to anticipate their emergence or aggravation. The team can then implement strategies to deal with them. Ethicists sometimes call this preventive ethics. As well as thwarting ethical problems, it can reduce complaints and lawsuits. It can improve the patient's experience and management and can help clinicians feel that they are providing ethically appropriate care. In the case above, the first 'ethics' task is to discuss the issue of confidentiality with the patient.

The checklist should be concise and easy to understand (there may be dozens of patients to consider that morning), and the categories should capture the ethical issues most common in hospital medicine. The section would appear after the social or family history. In the case of the patient with HIV, such an ethics checklist might look like the one below. In practice, the presenter might say, "With regard to ethical issues, patient confidentiality and disclosure of HIV status to the wife and girlfriend, because of the risk of HIV transmission, are notable. The patient's views on disclosure are not known."

The checklist serves as a prompt to help clinicians confront the ethical issues. Once these are identified, the team can decide how to address them. Depending on the complexity of the problems, they may handle them locally, consult a hospital ethicist (if available, which is unlikely in the UK but more so in North America), or refer the case to the clinical ethics committee. Often the presenter will simply say that there are no notable ethical issues. Completing the checklist should seldom take longer than 30 seconds, and the time spent doing so may well be saved later.

Recently a colleague and I went on rounds in an intensive care unit. One of the doctors was presenting the patient: a demented man who was terminally ill. The team spent 20 minutes discussing the patient's management. As the senior physician was putting the final touches to the chart, my colleague asked whether the patient had an advance directive. The nurse leafed through the voluminous notes and found an advance directive. It stated that in the event of an irreversible, end-stage condition the patient wanted comfort care only – no ventilation or other life-sustaining measures. The management plan was swiftly changed.

Without my colleague's intervention the patient would have continued to be treated against his previously expressed wishes. The checklist would probably have prevented the error. The presenter might say: "In terms of ethical issues, the patient has a detailed advanced directive expressing a refusal of life sustaining treatment in end-stage conditions. The goal of care should thus be reconsidered, with limitation of treatment, including DNAR [do not attempt resuscitation]."

This is the ethics equivalent of the World Health

Organization's surgical checklist. Like its surgical counterpart, it can prevent mistakes. It too takes only a handful of seconds. It too forces the healthcare team to acknowledge explicitly aspects that may be overlooked. Washington Hospital Center, in the District of Columbia, has used the checklist. So too has the University of Sheffield as a tool for teaching medical students about ethics.

Washington Hospital Center's ethics checklist:

Patient's wishes unclear/ refusal of treatment
Questionable capacity to consent to, or refuse treatment
Disagreement involving relatives/ surrogate/ caregivers
End-of-life (adv dir/ POA, DNR/ AND, withdraw/ withold Rx)
Goal of care clarification/ appropriateness of current treatment
Confidentiality/ disclosure
Resource or fairness issue
Other (please note)
No notable ethical issues

To the sceptics I ask this question: if you were a patient, would you prefer your medical team to use an ethics checklist?

Having seen many ethical mishaps in hospitals, I know what my answer would be.

WHEN DOCTORS DECEIVE EACH OTHER

In my mid-20s I spent 3 years of my life pondering the following question: "Can doctors ever justifiably deceive their patients?" The answer, in a word, was yes. Contrary to professional guidelines and modern codes of ethics, I argued that benevolent deception by doctors is, on rare occasions, morally permissible. Many readers were not amused. Some pointed to the guidance of the General Medical Council, which states that one of the cardinal duties of a doctor is to "be honest and open and act with integrity." Readers will not be amused at this chapter either, for it addresses a delicate issue seldom raised in the literature: doctors deceiving each other. To my deception-sensitive eyes, there is an elephant in the hospital and, following the advice of the late Professor Randy Pausch, I shall introduce it.

A doctor needs a computed tomography (CT) scan for his patient. To obtain the scan in good time he feigns concern about a possible pulmonary embolus on the radiology request form. He is also aware that, in the eyes of his consultant, a measure of his competence is how promptly and reliably he can obtain scans. Under interrogation by the radiologist, the doctor embellishes the truth to justify the urgency. An honest approach may have delayed matters. When asked about this practice the answer is usually pragmatic: "Everybody else is doing it." Such widespread manipulation creates a tension between two fundamental duties: the duty to be honest to colleagues and the duty to make the care of your own patient your first concern.

The embellishment to the radiologist may improve that particular patient's care, but it can also result in an unjust prioritisation of scans, with potential harm to other patients. The biased presentation can also lead radiologists to interpret the scans inaccurately, and this in turn can lead the referring doctor to provide needless and risky interventions. Leslie and colleagues have shown that inexact clinical information can adversely affect the computed tomography reports of consultant radiologists. What untold harm is caused by this deception? Is the system in a state of satisfactory equilibrium, or should it be changed? If the latter, how should we change it?

Some doctors use a similar strategy to get a patient seen at an emergency clinic or admitted to a particular ward. A doctor on a general ward calls the intensive treatment registrar and lies about the patient's previous quality of life to boost the probability of admission. It is only when the patient arrives on the ward that the truth emerges. Another doctor uses the same tactic to persuade surgeons to operate on a desperate patient. Once again, this may lead to injustice. The patients in greatest medical need may not get the appropriate care.

And surgeons too can indulge in a spot of deception, telling the anaesthetist that the case will take only 30 minutes when it will clearly take longer, or that an operation will be straightforward when it probably will not. In anaesthesia, an occasional deception occurs when the surgeon, struggling to operate during a difficult case, asks the anaesthetist to administer more muscle relaxant. The anaesthetist, whose monitoring tells him that paralysis is adequate, acquiesces and injects a dose of saline.

If failing to report something when there is a professional duty to do so constitutes deception by omission, then many doctors deceive occupational health staff by concealing their needlestick injuries. Out of fear or solidarity, doctors may also cover up a colleague's mistake. Many frustrated doctors have double checked, time and again, the actions of a substandard colleague, wondering whether a job was done properly. When teaching junior doctors I have been consistently surprised by how the efforts of some brave soul to report an incompetent colleague to seniors have been quashed. The 'dangerous colleague' question is commonly asked at interviews for membership examinations to the Royal Colleges, but when acted on in practice the outcome can be quite different. Another deception occurs when a trainee makes up a test result to save face in front of a consultant ("blood test X was normal").

Then there are those less serious deceptions to justify an absence from work or to provide a compelling reason to swap a shift with a colleague. The doctor, asked if he can cover a sick colleague, may claim to be at the other end of the country when he is nearby. He may say he is too drunk to work the next day when he is sober. He may make up all sorts of excuses.

There are those deceptions on job application forms, perhaps exaggerating a position of responsibility or inventing some audit that will tick an all-important box; and those in the realm of publications, such as adding the name of non-contributing colleagues to articles before submission.

Many years ago, one of my medical students conducted an exploratory study on doctors deceiving doctors. It was geographically diverse and anonymous. The research ethics committee got nervous. I called the General Medical Council, which reassured me and the committee that it could not discipline the respondents if the survey was anonymous. Still, the response rate was extremely low, indicating perhaps that it is an issue that many doctors would rather not discuss, even anonymously. Fifteen of the 23 respondents said they had deceived colleagues.

So, what should we make of all this? The immediate answer is that we should look at the situation more closely rather than avert our eyes. The focus has hitherto been on doctors deceiving patients and, to a much lesser extent, patients deceiving doctors. Despite the disapproving glares of unamused colleagues, we need also to be 'honest and open' about the deceptions that occur between clinicians so that we can identify why they occur. Only then can we distinguish between those that are unjustified and need to be eliminated and those, if any, that are permitted.

THE LAWYER'S BRIEF ON ETHICS

In August 2009 I resigned from my position as an academic medical ethicist to train as a barrister. Upon hearing of my change a friend quipped, "Ah, you've given up ethics to be a lawyer." To many people 'ethics' and 'lawyers' are like oil and water. In the popular perception, lawyers have no scruples and earn vast sums of money, even defending murderers, rapists, and paedophiles. In the context of medicine they sue well-meaning clinicians and attempt deviously to undermine the authority of esteemed consultants in cross examination. Eager was I, then, to find out whether ethics had a place in a lawyer's training.

There was not a drop of teaching of ethics in my first year of law, the so-called 'conversion' year. We were taught to change our way of thinking from that of a layperson ("That's jolly unfair!") to that of a lawyer ("Is there a wrongful act in law?"). We were taught the law from an academic perspective: imagine a surgeon who leaves a swab in a patient's abdomen, or a general practitioner who fails to diagnose a malignant melanoma; what must you prove to determine whether the clinician is liable in negligence?

My first contact with ethics came towards the

end of the first year, during the dreaded interviews for 'pupillage'. Pupillage refers to the first year in a barrister's career. Nearly every interview contained a question about ethics. You are defending an elderly woman charged with driving under the influence. She has told you in conference – a private meeting – that she drinks no alcohol. On the morning of the trial you notice her outside the court room, suspiciously sipping a bottle wrapped in a brown paper bag. What do you do? Or, you are defending an alleged rapist who tells you, again in conference, that he did commit the offence but that he nonetheless wants to plead not guilty. Another client assures you of his innocence but insists on pleading guilty to benefit from a reduced sentence.

The second year is the vocational part of the course. Reality, in the form of a client, has appeared on the scene, and the client cares not a jot for arcane legal debates. Clients want to know whether they will win their case, or how much money they can get, or whether they will go to jail, or whether they can visit their children. And with reality comes ethics.

All aspiring barristers must now pass an ethics exam. It is not possible to qualify as a barrister without obtaining at least 60%. Will medical schools follow suit and set a separate ethics exam, rather than the odd question interspersed here and there? It would heighten the status of ethics in the curriculum, although it can hardly be denied that medical students are already overexamined.

There are clear parallels between legal and medical

ethics. Paragraph 303 of the Bar Code of Conduct states that a barrister must "promote and protect fearlessly and by all proper and lawful means the lay client's best interests." Like doctors and their competent patients, it is ultimately up to the client to decide what course of action to take, even if the barrister considers it morally wrong or foolish. This is, in effect, respect for the client's autonomy. If the self-confessed rapist wants to plead not guilty and cannot be persuaded to do otherwise, then the barrister must defend him. The burden of proof is on the prosecution to prove guilt; the barrister, however, will not be permitted to mislead the judge or jury by stating expressly that the client is innocent.

The 'cab rank' rule is neatly explained by Horace Rumpole, the memorable barrister in John Mortimer's novels. "I'm a black taxi, plying for hire," bellows Rumpole. "I'm bound to accept anyone, however repulsive, who waves me down and asks for a lift." Barristers must accept any case that comes their way, not just those that are considered morally worthy. They cannot pick and choose. Doctors too have a cab rank rule. They cannot usually refuse to treat patients because they find them morally objectionable. Any visible injection of moral judgment in the doctor–patient relationship would be a backward step. Doctors, like lawyers, are not moral judges.

Confidentiality, known as legal professional privilege, is also sacrosanct, perhaps more so than in the doctor–patient relationship. Without the client's permission the barrister will not tell a soul that the client has knowingly built an extension on a neighbour's land or confessed to killing a lover. As well as bolstering trust, this promise of silence allows clients to talk honestly with their lawyer, and this in turn enables the lawyer to give appropriate advice. Similar reasoning underpins the duty of confidentiality on doctors: without it, patients may hold back information that could otherwise assist the doctor in making a diagnosis.

As in medicine, I wonder to what extent the lofty tenets of the barristers' code of ethics are applied in practice. Doubtless the extent to which they are respected depends on the individual practitioner. At law school we are constantly reminded that lawyers, like doctors, can be sued for negligence. Some lawyers specialise in suing other lawyers. The Bar Standards Board has disciplinary hearings to handle complaints against barristers. "Violate the code and kiss goodbye to your career" is the barely disguised message. Yet the emphasis is in the wrong place. The motivation to be ethical should be rooted not in the fear of getting into trouble but in the belief that a good lawyer, like a good doctor, is necessarily an ethical one.

TEACHING MEDICAL ETHICS: USEFUL OR USELESS?

Probably for the first time in history, UK-trained doctors at all levels, and in all specialties, now receive formal ethics training at medical school. This raises an important but uncomfortable question for those who teach the subject: has it made any difference? If not, should we replace it with another course on pharmacology, clinical skills, or the interpretation of scans?

An 'ethics' sceptic will point to the vast increase in numbers of complaints against doctors to the UK General Medical Council in the past 10 years and the growth of clinical negligence claims in that same period. The annual cash spending for clinical negligence cases against NHS Trusts rose from £0.5 billion in 2006 to £1.7 billion in 2016. The number of successful clinical negligence claims leading to an award of damages went from 2,800 to 7,300. More ethics, more complaints and law suits, and less money to deliver healthcare to patients.

This sceptic may say that any improvement in 'ethics' arises not from any teaching in medical ethics but from changes in the law, such as the case of **Montgomery** for consent, **Tracey** for "Do not attempt cardiopulmonary resuscitation", and the statutory duty of candour for truth-telling and honesty. In fact, the sceptic may add, the existence of these cases and the very need for a statutory duty of candour indicate that ethics training has made little difference to actual practice.

Using anecdotal evidence, the sceptic will point to the low status of the subject among most medical students, who deem it "irrelevant", "impractical", "unclear".

In response, the ethics supporter would seek to dissociate the increase in complaints and litigation from the general levels of ethical behaviour, pointing to changing expectations among patients and relatives, the role of the media (including social media) in encouraging complaints, rapacious lawyers, and a greater awareness of complaint processes and the role of the GMC. There is no obvious link between the rising number of complaints and falling standards of clinical or ethical competence, the supporter would say.

Nor does the supposed unpopularity of ethics among medical students indicate a lack of value. Many doctors say that it is only once they start working that they appreciate the subject's relevance. The ethically trained doctor possesses the tools to escape from the occupational hazard that is clinical myopia.

The answer, of course, is that we do not know whether teaching ethics to medical students makes any long-term difference to their clinical practice. The effects of the teaching may impinge positively on a student's outlook, attitude, or character but may not be tangible or measurable. If a doctor who would otherwise have seen a dying patient for a few seconds before moving on decides out of kindness and compassion to stay a little longer with the patient, to comfort and reassure, is this attributable to ethics teaching at medical school, the doctor's upbringing, a natural disposition, or last night's episode of *Casualty*? It is too complex a situation to draw out cause and effect.

The bioethicist Judith Andre wrote that teaching ethics is "fundamentally an act of hope." We usually have no idea whether such teaching matters. No doubt skewed by the incessant stream of clinical negligence contained in my cases, I have become less certain over time of the effect of ethics teaching at medical school on the future behaviour of doctors, especially if it is delivered in the early years.

The bulk of this teaching should take place after qualification, in the clinical setting. Before then, most students care about one thing only: passing exams.

Yet, the very presence of ethics in the curriculum is important. It sends a message that ethics is an intrinsic and valued part of medical practice. The teaching of ethics, even if its worth can't be proved, is consistent with common sense and may reassure members of the public that the medical profession, for all the changes since the oath of Hippocrates, has not lost its moral compass.

THE ART OF MEDICAL ETHICS

THE MOMENT OF TRUTH

Edmund Pellegrino, a professor of medicine and a giant of medical ethics, once said that for the clinician the "moment of truth may come at three in the morning, when no one is watching." This prompted me to ponder on "the moment of truth". What is it? And can we prepare for it?

The moment of truth is a bullfighting term. The "hora de verdad" refers to the moment when the matador entices the bull with the 'muleta' (the red cape draped over a stick) and, with the precision of the anaesthetist hitting the epidural space in an obese patient, plunges the sword into the bull's neck for the kill. If he thrusts the sword at a slight angle he will sever the aorta and the bull will die in seconds. If the matador misses, his body is exposed to the sharp horns of the frenzied animal.

We encounter a moment of truth when we are put to the test, and how we respond becomes a measure of our worth. Sometimes, as in an acute emergency, the moment of truth is clear: the patient is hypoxic, oropharyngeal visibility is poor from the blood and swelling of trauma, and the tube must go in immediately. At other times, especially with patients with more chronic illness, the moment of truth is identified only retrospectively. A doctor may realise too late that he or she omitted something that could have prevented a poor outcome, such as the radiologist who realises that he or she missed a lesion on the X-ray picture.

The moment of truth can involve physical actions, as in the difficult intubation; decisions, as with the surgeon contemplating whether to operate; or attitudes to events or circumstances.

The 'truth' in the phrase "the moment of truth" can refer to true skill, true merit, or true strength of character. We can prepare by honing our technical competencies. The cardiothoracic surgeon Fyodor Uglov, famous for his technique, sutured 400 rubber gloves before performing anastomoses on patients. Alone, at 3 in the morning, the well prepared trainee can insert that all-important central line in the patient with a sudden onset of severe sepsis. It is this fear of encountering the moment of truth that, at least in part, explains why some junior doctors look on the night shift with dread.

We can work on developing our character, putting ourselves in situations in which we can learn to exercise virtues such as courage, kindness, and wisdom. This may require us to seek new experiences and step outside our comfort zone.

A turning point in my development as a medical ethicist was on hearing a song, *Moi mes souliers*, by the Canadian singer Félix Leclerc. It is about a man's travels and adventures, from school to war, through fields of mud, through countless villages and streams. The final stanza, loosely translated, goes: "Heaven, my friends, is not the place for polished shoes. So if you seek forgiveness, hurry and get your shoes dirty." As I could see my own reflection in my shoes, I travelled to various hospitals around the world to get them dirty.

Alone, at 3 in the morning, the trainee with dirty shoes can then decide to reassure a frightened patient when it would be easy to pretend not to notice. However, even with the cultivation of skill and virtue, it is impossible to prepare fully for some moments of truth, those monumental ones defined by their life-changing nature.

Moments of truth reveal something fundamental about ourselves, and as such they represent an opportunity for self improvement. They are perhaps unique to humans. The charging bull cannot conceive of a moment of truth. Only the matador can experience it, thinking to himself, as he sees the saliva flying from the charging animal's mouth, "This is it." For Pellegrino and many medical ethicists who call themselves 'virtue theorists', the focus of medical ethics should not be on what is the right or wrong action but on developing the character of the clinician.

Respected clinicians on the wards and in the GP's surgery have a much greater influence in the development of virtue in students than my colleagues and I do in the classroom. It is difficult to teach courage or integrity in a packed lecture theatre. Virtues in medicine are learnt most effectively by watching and learning from clinicians who act virtuously. Ideally the bulk of medical ethics should be taught on the wards, for ethical decisions in clinical medicine are made under conditions that cannot be recreated in a classroom.

Repeated, realistic exposure is the key to good ethical training. After all, it is in the arena – with the cheering crowd, blistering heat, dazzling sun, swirling sand, and raging bull – that matadors learn the essence of their art.

HOW TO THINK LIKE AN ETHICIST

Structure. That is the key. Structure. Did John steal the stethoscope? Go through each of the five components of theft: appropriation, of property, belonging to another, dishonestly, with the intention to permanently deprive. If a single element is missing, there is no theft. Was Jane negligent when she failed to intubate the young child? Go through the elements of negligence: loss, duty of care, standard of care, breach, causation, and remoteness. Throughout the last year at law school we were told to "think like lawyers". We had to lose the deep-rooted instinct to judge the morality of a person's act and replace it with a dispassionate legal dissection of the facts at hand.

When training in medical ethics I was never told to "think like an ethicist". There is no universally accepted way to do ethics, and at times the words from a Dilbert comic strip posted on the notice board of a bioethics department ring worryingly true. Having received the advice he wanted to hear, Dilbert muses that "90% of happiness is finding the right ethicist."

If I were asked to train readers to be medical ethicists (the kind that I would like my doctor to consult if morally perplexed), structure would feature early in the syllabus. The method would be the 'four quadrants' approach, developed by the Americans Albert Jonsen, Mark Siegler, and William Winslade in the early 1980s. A brief demonstration (which is based on an example given in Jonsen and colleagues' book) follows.

Lucy is an 8-year-old girl with a diagnosis of acute myeloid leukaemia. Three months after a course of chemotherapy she relapsed. A transplantation of bone marrow from her older sister was performed. Again, she soon relapsed. Although the oncologist told Lucy's parents that further chemotherapy would provide scant benefit, they insisted on more. The medical team attempted a course of experimental chemotherapy, which unfortunately did not slow the progress of the disease. Lucy, a once cheerful patient, is now despondent. She asks, "Why must I keep doing this?"

The temptation to 'jump in' with gut reactions must be resisted. Good ethics starts with good facts. The first quadrant of our analysis, therefore, is clinical indications. What is Lucy's likely prognosis? What is the treatment goal, and how likely are we to attain it? If the proposed treatment does not work, what is plan B? This quadrant clarifies the medical situation and seeks to highlight the harm and benefits of any proposed intervention. Doctors should feel on familiar territory here. The ideal scenario is that the medical team, after reviewing the situation, agrees on the clinical 'ought'. Of course, in reality, the medical situation may be messy, with various unknowns and disagreements.

Once the medical indications are clear – or as clear as they can be – the next quadrant looks at the patient's preferences. Is Lucy competent to take part in decisions about her care? If so, has she been informed of the situation, and what are her thoughts on the matter? Lucy's remark suggests that someone needs to talk to her about her future care. Keeping her in the dark runs counter to the principle of respect for autonomy and may lead Lucy to feel isolated or abandoned. If dealing with an incompetent adult we would consider prior preferences, including any advance statements.

Next, we consider the third quadrant: quality of life. What will the effect of any proposed intervention be on Lucy's quality of life? How will further aggressive treatment, for example, affect her mental, physical, and social wellbeing? Again, there is no certainty in this assessment, but it is an important factor in deciding what is in Lucy's best interest. An intervention may be medically indicated because it will prolong life. This quadrant will question the value of such an extension. For Lucy, palliative care may be more appropriate.

Then we turn to the final quadrant: contextual features. This is a hotch-potch category, containing all other relevant factors. In Lucy's case, we would explore the views and feelings of her parents and sister and any underlying religious or cultural issues. Clinicians, too, have prejudices and biases that can affect their decision-making, whether they are based on religion, past experience, self interest, or hospital politics. This is also the place to consider the delicate issue of resource allocation and any pertinent legal rules or professional guidelines.

That, in a nutshell, is the four quadrants approach: start with clinical indications and move on to examine patient preferences, then quality of life, and finally contextual features. It is no panacea, however. Sound judgment and an open mind are needed to balance the various considerations raised in the analysis. A solution will not always emerge from the foggy moral landscape; but more often than not it will clear some of the haze and expose the mines strewn along the way. Like any skill, it gets easier with practice.

In the 13th century the surgeon Lanfranc wrote that "no one can be a good physician who has no idea of surgical operations, and a surgeon is nothing if ignorant of medicine." Today, physicians and surgeons operate in a morally laden clinical environment, and neither group can be truly at ease without a method to examine the ethical issues in their practice. The four quadrants of ethics should be as familiar to doctors as the four quadrants of the abdomen.

BATTLING PROFESSOR PINKER

When I was an undergraduate student in linguistics in the 1990s, Professor Steven Pinker was a living legend in the field. In August 2015, he strayed beyond his area of expertise.

Before scientists can conduct research on human beings, they often need approval from research ethics committees or, in North America, Institutional Review Boards. So, if scientists at British American Tobacco want to investigate the effect of a new tobacco product on people's lungs, they would need permission from a research ethics committee. If scientists from the University of Oxford want to test a new anti-malaria vaccine on students, they would also need ethics approval.

In an Opinion piece in the *Boston Globe*, Professor Pinker made the surprising suggestion that the primary moral goal of bioethics – by that he means ethicists and research ethics committees – should be to "get out of the way". "A truly ethical bioethics," he argued, "should not bog down research in red tape, moratoria or threats of prosecution."

This bold assertion no doubt echoes the thoughts of many scientists whose research requires the approval of an ethics review committee before springing to life. As a PhD student many years ago, I experienced first-hand the frustrations of the tedious review process. I spent hours drafting the protocol and revisions and responding to the committee's questions, time I would have preferred to spend conducting research. While a popular sentiment, getting out of the way is not the goal of bioethics.

The goal of bioethics is to allow potentially beneficial research while ensuring that the risk of harm to participants and others is proportionate, reduced to the lowest practicable level, and within morally acceptable limits. The risk of harm can never be eliminated, but it can usually be reduced with minimal effort or cost. It may be as simple as testing a new piece of equipment one more time in a laboratory before attaching it to a human for testing.

At times, researchers – who in their enthusiasm may not have considered the risks of harm as carefully as an impartial judge – underestimate or overlook the potential harm to others. In those situations, an ethics committee should 'get in the way', point out the problems, and if possible suggest ways of surmounting them. Speaking from personal experience, no ethics committee wants a death under its watch. Academic bioethicists may talk of 'dignity', 'sacredness', and other nebulous notions in scholarly documents but, in the front line of ethical decision-making, the focus is on the very real physical and psychological harm that may befall participants.

Bioethics is not opposed to research and progress.

The search for solutions to the suffering of humankind is, in itself, a moral imperative, but misguided attempts to help can – and have – lead to incalculable harm. Examples of harmful research are many. A notable example is the Tuskegee experiment in Alabama, in which poor black men with syphilis were observed from 1932 to 1972 to understand the natural progression of the disease. When effective drugs (penicillin) became available in the 1940s, the study continued without offering the treatment, or even information about the treatment, to the participants.

Some of these examples, including the Tuskegee study, were the triggers to the safeguards, principles, codes, and declarations that pertain to contemporary biomedical research.

Knowing what we know about human nature, to let researchers evaluate the ethics of their own research is akin to the police judging other policemen, or doctors judging other doctors. Virtually everyone would, in good faith but quite wrongly, consider their research ethically exemplary.

Professor Pinker worries about the threat of prosecution as an obstacle, but it is a legitimate concern. What sensible researcher would not want to know about the risk of being sued? The level and likelihood of risk are best assessed by lawyers, but the matter should be raised by an ethics review committee. Review by a committee may itself reduce the risk of litigation. Professor Pinker sees ethics committees as adversaries of researchers whereas, in fact, they strive to assist them rather than finding fault for its own sake. They are on the same team, or at least they should be.

Bioethics suffers from an image problem. Bioethicists are viewed by some researchers as the 'ethics police', as legislators and enforcers of their own moral law. Admittedly, some bioethicists suffer from a kind of ethical hypochondria, prone to catastrophic thinking, the belief that every protocol or project is plagued with ethical boils. Just as surgeons have a natural inclination to operate and lawyers tend to see the 'worst-case scenario', bioethicists can see ethical problems that are too remote and over-stress their significance.

There are, without doubt, members of bioethics committees whose disposition and judgment are incompatible with their membership. I have witnessed ugly scenes when members of a research ethics committee have questioned researchers with the venom of a cross-examination in a criminal trial, and when researchers have failed to give the process of ethical review the necessary attention, turning up to the meeting unprepared. There are good and bad researchers, and so too bioethicists.

The recruitment, experience, and training of members of ethics committees are legitimate concerns; perhaps more members should have direct experience of the type of research they are reviewing.

The idea that research that has the potential to cause harm should be subject to ethical review should not be controversial in the 21st century. The words "this project has been reviewed and approved by the Research Ethics

Committee" offers some reassurance that the welfare of participants has been duly considered. The thought of biomedical research without ethical review is a frightening one.

ON MORAL VISION

Over a beer Jim celebrates his first draw against an international chess master, the rank just below the coveted title of grandmaster (GM). I joke that GMs are next on the menu. "No," he says, "these guys see things on the board which us mortals can't see."

A magician asks a spectator to name any playing card. The five of hearts. The magician opens his wallet, then the zipped compartment within, and pulls out the chosen card. After the show 3 magicians search in vain for a solution. An experienced magician joins the group and immediately suggests an ingenious and plausible method.

Harvey Cushing, in one of his essays, wrote of a patient who was admitted to hospital with an unexplained fever. Various tests were done: blood, urine, sputum, stool, cerebrospinal fluid. Specialists were called in. Meanwhile the fever continued. A country doctor who was visiting the hospital walked past the patient's bed and said, "I am surprised to see that you still have an occasional case of typhoid fever in your neighborhood."

In each of these vignettes one individual is blessed with greater vision than the rest. Each shares the ability to identify salient features, a meaningful pattern, or a constellation of signs and symptoms, and to derive a hypothesis or an appropriate plan of action. They have vision. In the realm of ethics we talk of moral vision or moral perception. Like the mythical hundred-eyed giant Argus, whose eyes now adorn the tail of the peacock, a morally perceptive person sees ethical aspects of a situation that may not be readily apparent to others.

After several failed attempts to lose weight, Gloria, a morbidly obese 44-year-old woman, was eligible for gastric bypass surgery. As she had had an open cholecystectomy previously, she was scheduled for an open procedure. Her hypertension and diabetes were well controlled, and Gloria told her doctor that she was looking forward to caring for her disabled son.

At this point the doctor could have sent her to the operating theatre and moved on to the next patient on his list. Instead, concerned by that last statement, he asked her about her son. He was in the final stages of muscular dystrophy. Gloria's alcoholic husband was violent and unhelpful. She stayed with him only for financial reasons to support her disabled son and young daughter. After discussing the likely effect of the operation on her ability to care for the children, Gloria postponed the procedure. "They need me now more than ever," she observed.

The doctor displayed moral perception by thinking beyond surgical eligibility and considering the suitability of the procedure for this individual in this situation at this time. Picking up on an important cue, the doctor saw the patient within a broader social context.

The antithesis of moral vision is moral blindness. The morally blind person fails to see the ethically problematic nature of a situation. In 2003 a study in the *BMJ* showed that almost a quarter of intimate examinations of anaesthetised patients by medical students were performed without consent. In an interview one fourth year student said, "I was told in the second year that the best way to learn to do PRs [rectal examinations] was when the patient was under anaesthetic. That way they would never know." A myopic cyclops, this student: the moral issue does not even appear on his radar. The patient seems little more than an instrument for his own clinical development.

Improving moral vision should be the first step in the teaching of ethics in medicine, for sophisticated reasoning is useless without the moral vision needed to trigger the reasoning process. A host of obstacles – whether due to moral ignorance or naivety, to the clinical mindset, with its emphasis on physiology and hard science, or to the many pressures and distractions on the ward – can prevent students from seeing clearly.

Judith Andre, a US bioethicist, believes that one of the greatest obstacles is lack of time. When time is short, ethical issues are missed. (And so are clinical issues; recall Osler's famous words: "Hurry is the devil. More people are killed by hurry than by disease.") Patients may even be seen as 'consumers of time' who impede other priorities. Time is also essential for reflection, an activity central to moral growth.

Although junior doctors, who are forced to write

reflective pieces as part of their training, may growl at the sight of the word, reflection is, for Andre, "the stage which allows half-perceived problems to be fully seen." One obvious requirement to improve moral acuity, then, is to give students and clinicians time to reflect on their experiences and on how their background, colleagues, surroundings, institution, and society shape their views on medicine, bringing some aspects into focus and pushing others out of sight.

If we can provide this all-important time for reflection (however difficult this may be), if we can show in our teaching how moral choices (such as those involving futility and best interests – see the next two chapters) may be disguised as purely medical choices, if we can encourage clinicians on the wards to instruct and inspire their juniors through their own attitudes and behaviours, and if we can give students the confidence to speak up and ask questions when in moral doubt, then more Arguses and fewer cyclopses will inhabit the ethical landscape of the clinic.

THE SLIPPERINESS OF FUTILITY

He was shot in the back. The surgeons could not save him. He lay in bed, unconscious, his life ebbing away as blood trickled down tubes to large jars at the base of his bed. As cardiopulmonary resuscitation would have been futile, we wrote a *Do Not Attempt Resuscitation* order. The case reminded me of the etymology of the word 'futile'. 'Futilis', in Latin, means 'leaky'. The patient was leaking blood from various wounds, and nothing could stop it.

At an examiners' meeting, a professor of surgery admitted that he would have got the ethics question wrong. The question concerned the definition of futility. "So how would you define futility?" I asked. He paused and, in a Humpty Dumpty way, answered: "Something is futile if I say it is." This remark highlights the slipperiness and subjectivity of the term 'futile'. Yet, in the clinical front line, futility, coated with a veneer of objectivity, is often used as a moral trump card, a dismissive pronouncement to end all discussion: "I'm sorry. We're stopping aggressive care. It's futile."

Psychiatrists must sigh in frustration when asked if a patient has capacity. The capacity to decide what? Similarly, futility is not free-floating but linked to a specific goal. Prescribing antibiotics for a viral illness is physiologically futile but if the doctor's goal is to leave the surgery in time for the first aria in *Don Giovanni*, then it is not (although this would still be a breach of the duty of care!). Futility, then, is goal-specific, and when you next hear doctors say that such-and-such is futile, you can surprise them and ask "futile with respect to what?".

When teaching the subject to medical students, I shuffle a pack of playing cards, select a card at random, and ask if it is futile for them to guess the identity of the card. Some say yes, others say no, and once in a blue moon a statistically minded student will ask if the two jokers are included in the pack. Never is there unanimous agreement. The point of the exercise is to illustrate the variability of our quantitative assessment of futility. In the literature, some scholars have suggested that an intervention is futile if it has not worked in the last hundred cases. Under that definition, guessing the card would not be quantitatively futile. Even if we accept this somewhat arbitrary 'last hundred times' rule, in practice the problem is that it is rarely possible to know whether an intervention has worked the last hundred times, especially as no two cases are identical.

The students who believe in the futility of naming the card still venture a guess if tempted by a £50 cash prize. The perceived futility of the exercise does not translate into a refusal to try. The reason is that there is no cost associated with the guess. The benefit is potentially significant and the cost minimal. As Kite and Wilkinson point out, sometimes the reason why clinicians withhold or withdraw an intervention is not because it probably won't fulfil its purpose, but because it will cause harm or deprive others of benefit. An intervention can be simultaneously futile, harmful, and wasteful.

One of the saddest cases I have seen involved a woman so viciously mauled by dogs that she was left in a vegetative state. When considering her resuscitation status, one of the doctors stated that she should not be resuscitated on the grounds of futility. When probed further, it emerged that the doctor believed the patient's quality of life was so awful that CPR was not medically indicated. This is another type of futility: qualitative futility. It is based on a subjective evaluation of whether the goal of the intervention is worthwhile.

While ethically aware readers need not be familiar with the vast literature on the concept of futility, they might wish to remember the following points:

1. Futility is goal-specific.
2. **Physiological futility** is when the proposed intervention cannot physiologically achieve the desired effect. It is the most objective type of futility judgment.
3. **Quantitative futility** is when the proposed intervention is highly unlikely to achieve the desired effect.
4. **Qualitative futility** is when the proposed intervention, if successful, will probably produce such a poor outcome that it is deemed best not to attempt it.

When using the term, clinicians may be referring to several types of futility, for example that an intervention is highly unlikely to achieve the goal (quantitative futility) *and* that the goal itself is undesirable (qualitative futility). As futility is so rhetorically powerful and semantically fuzzy, doctors may find it helpful to distinguish between physiological, quantitative, and qualitative futility. This classification reveals that a futility call, far from being objective, can be coloured by the values of the person making the call. Like 'best interests', 'futility' exudes a confident air of objectivity while concealing value judgments.

I conclude this chapter on a practical note. Clinicians should be wary of using 'futile' in front of patients and relatives. As Jonsen, Siegler, and Winslade propose, it may be better to think in terms of proportionality, or "the balance of expected benefits over burdens imposed by continued interventions." Furthermore, 'futile' suggests that nothing can be done. Recall the ancient medical wisdom: "To cure, sometimes. To relieve, often. To comfort, always." There is always something to be done.

CLARIFYING BEST INTERESTS

If from the lamp emerged a bioethics genie who granted me only one wish, I would ask for the ability to determine what is in the best interests of a particular individual. With such insight I would resolve many of the thorniest dilemmas in clinical ethics, discerning immediately what is best for the patient. Should we withhold treatment from this severely disabled neonate? Should we repeatedly inform this woman with Alzheimer's disease that her husband died 10 years ago? Should we respect the confidentiality of this sexually active 14-year-old girl?

Nowadays it is almost trite to say that 'best interests' is a broader term than 'medical best interests'. While important, health is one value among others that may, on occasion, be offset by those others. Hence a bon vivant might accept the life shortening effects of eating full fat brie daily in exchange for the pleasure he derives from it. Overall best interests may legitimately differ from medical best interests, and the two should not be confused.

The philosopher Ronald Dworkin makes another useful distinction: between experiential interests and critical interests. Experiential interests concern our sensations of pain and pleasure. I have experiential interests in playing squash, performing magic, and writing this book. Under this conception, it makes no sense to talk of the experiential interests of patients in a persistent vegetative state. They have no such interests.

They do, however, have critical interests. These concern the sort of things that give meaning to our lives, that ultimately determine whether our lives are going well or badly. Friendship, the wellbeing of loved ones, and the respect of others are examples of critical interests. These can be frustrated or satisfied even in the absence of consciousness. Spreading malicious rumours behind someone's back can harm their critical interests even if that person never finds out; so too can failing to discharge a promise to hand over a dead person's savings to her children. Why? Because most people have critical interests in maintaining a good reputation and helping their family to flourish.

The existence of critical interests explains why clinicians should attempt to uncover patients' past and present wishes, either by consulting the patients themselves (or their relatives) or from written documents such as advanced statements. What things are important to this person? How can we respect his or her critical values in our clinical management? To paraphrase Professor Gillon, the trick is not to put ourselves in the patient's shoes, but to imagine what it is like for the patient to be in his or her shoes. This requires an appreciation of that person's experiential and critical interests. When patients are unable to make their own decisions, doctors should, on legal and ethical grounds, act in their best interests.

However, even when patients are autonomous most doctors strive to do their best for their patients. In his book *Resolving Ethical Dilemmas* Bernard Lo offers a strategy to promote a competent patient's best interests. This strategy could also be used by relatives and loved ones.

Firstly, try to understand the patient's perspective ("What worries you most about this illness/treatment/ operation?"). Secondly, address any concerns and misunderstandings. This may be enough to resolve any initial disagreement about treatment. Thirdly, if appropriate, try to persuade the patient to accept medically indicated interventions. If persuasion is unsuccessful, negotiate a plan that is mutually acceptable to both parties. Try to find common ground, a compromise solution; give the patient more time or information to decide; and invite them to speak to another doctor or other patients with similar experiences. If this strategy fails, accept the patient's refusal. This approach aims to protect patients from seemingly unwise decisions, while respecting their autonomy.

As we have privileged access to our own interests, respecting a person's autonomy tends to benefit them. One of the greatest tragedies in medicine is when respecting a patient's autonomy has the opposite effect: when it goes against their critical interests. Although formally having capacity, we can sometimes be blind to our own good; thus the seropositive 25-year-old declines our outstretched hand at the edge of life's precipice, her judgment clouded by indifferent relatives and the short-lived experiential interests of illicit drugs. Her refusal to be treated signals a premature death. Such is the price of our liberal emphasis on respecting autonomy, whatever its undeniable benefits. Although it is legally obligatory in Britain and the United States, respecting a competent refusal of treatment is not always in the patient's best interests.

When there is no indication of a patient's values, how should we determine what is best? Clearly we should consider experiential interests. Yet critical interests also play a part, as all human beings share a common core of critical interests, such as the freedom from indignity.

The anencephalic baby with no prospects of a meaningful life has neither experiential nor critical interests in continued life. Where lies that indeterminate threshold below which attempting to prolong survival is no longer in a person's interests? This is where the genie's gift would be most helpful.

HARD CASES

EMBRACING THE ETHICALLY
COMPLICATED PATIENT

All clinicians are familiar with the medically complicated patient. Those patients have, for example, overlapping illnesses, complex manifestations of symptoms, or uncommon reactions to treatment. They fill the pages of medical journals as case reports. They are the subject of grand rounds and departmental meetings in hospitals.

Less celebrated is the ethically complicated patient. These are patients whose circumstances raise perplexing ethical questions for the healthcare team; and the care of such patients was the theme of the 2016 International Conference on Clinical Ethics Consultation, in Washington, DC.

The conference was an ethicist's dream but less so for a clinician, with case after case of conflicting values; tensions between patients, relatives, and medical teams; offensive, abusive, and racist patients; patients with borderline mental capacity; and uncertainties about 'best interests'.

We heard of a patient with an invariably fatal genetic disease who, after previous failed suicide attempts, told the medical team that she would kill herself once discharged. She had seen relatives succumb to the disease. Her psychiatrist said that she was depressed but had capacity. She was discharged and died shortly after. Should she have been discharged in those circumstances?

We heard of healthy but desperate patients who had asked for limb-lengthening procedures, now that the operation was safer than ever before. If a psychiatrist rules out any mental illness, should a surgeon agree to operate?

We heard the story of a 4-year-old boy with an incurable brainstem tumour. He developed right-sided weakness, gait disturbance, and speech problems. Then came wheezy breathing, headaches, swallowing problems, and decerebration cramps. He tried to talk but no one could understand him. He was sedated with midazolam, and the next week he underwent deep sedation with propofol. He remained unconscious until his death 10 days later. Was deep sedation ethically justified? How much information should doctors have given to this child before starting the deep sedation?

In each case the medical team called an ethicist to help them find an ethically acceptable solution or compromise. The ethicist talked to the stakeholders, identified their concerns, described the relevant ethical principles at play, and made recommendations to resolve the problem. Contrary to popular belief, clinical ethics is a practical discipline. It aims to be helpful, not obstructive.

Cases such as these highlight the gulf in clinical ethics support between large hospitals in the United States and

Canada, many of which have full-time ethicists, and the United Kingdom, with its sporadic use of committees. The UK trails far behind North America in the provision of ethics support for clinicians, as I have drawn attention to over the past decade. In the cases I've mentioned here most UK clinicians would have no access to on-site ethics support. They might 'muddle through', hoping not to miss anything of ethical or legal significance.

Whatever the availability of ethics support at their institution, clinicians should be as attentive to ethically complicated patients as to medically complicated ones. These patients should be the subject of as much thought and discussion. They should be discussed at multi-disciplinary team meetings, in grand rounds, and in case reports.

Albert Einstein reputedly said that in the middle of difficulty lies opportunity. The ethically complicated patient presents an opportunity to learn about whatever lies at the root of the complexity. Embracing these opportunities can improve the quality of patient care, lead to changes in practice and policy, and, if absorbed into the collective memory of the department, prevent the flaring up of ethical difficulties in the future.

LESSONS FROM THE ASHYA KING CASE

On 28th August 2014 the parents of 5-year-old Ashya King took him from Southampton General Hospital and boarded a ferry to France. He had been recovering from the removal of a medulloblastoma, a high-grade paediatric tumour.

Ashya's parents and doctors disagreed over his treatment. The parents sought proton beam therapy, arguing that it was less harmful than conventional radiotherapy. Peter Wilson, the lead paediatrician at the hospital, commented, "For this particular tumour, the reason why the proton beam was not deemed to be of any benefit is because you have to irradiate most of the brain and spine anyway." Proton beam therapy is not routinely provided on the NHS in England, although a small budget exists to take children abroad for treatment.

If a child lacks competence to make treatment decisions, the responsibility falls to the child's parents. Yet, the parents' right is not absolute. Where their instructions seem to conflict with the child's best interests, the doctors must seek the court's authority to override them, save for grave emergencies. A court can invoke its inherent jurisdiction under section 8 of the Children Act 1989 to make "specific issue orders" or "prohibited steps orders". In doing so, a judge will decide what is in the child's best interests.

In cases such as Ashya's, where there is a disagreement about treatment options, the onus is on the hospital to refer the matter to the courts. (Ashya's father claimed that the hospital's threat to apply for a court order prompted the family to remove Ashya.) That is the law. In practice, court orders can usually be averted by ongoing and open communication between the family and the medical team. We do not know what the nature of the communication was in Ashya's case; however, in general terms, the tendency to avoid difficult conversations must be resisted, and warning signs of a brewing disagreement – such as changes in the nature of a family's questions or their body language – must be acted on quickly.

Joseph Fins, the US bioethicist and professor of medicine, has written, "Too often, the culture of intensive care promotes and rewards diagnostic acumen and technical competence at the expense of communication. The result is that patients and family may feel bewildered and isolated at a time of crisis."

On discovering Ashya's absence, the hospital informed Hampshire police. The hospital feared that, if Ashya's nasogastric tube was displaced, feed could enter his lungs, with potentially fatal consequences. Without a gag reflex, he was at risk of choking. And the battery to his food pump was believed to be fast running out.

Ashya's parents had 'parental responsibility' when they removed him from hospital. It is therefore arguable that no permission from medical staff or the courts was needed. That the parents removed Ashya without telling anyone at the hospital, even if not legally obliged to do so, indicated the extent of the breakdown in trust between the family and the medical team.

Once alerted to the situation, the Crown Prosecution Service confirmed, on the basis of information from the hospital, that Ashya's life was at serious risk and that he needed urgent medical care. On 29th August 2014 Southampton Magistrates' Court issued a European arrest warrant. The basis on which it was issued was unclear, but Hampshire police said that it was "based around neglect".

Section 1 of the Children and Young Persons Act 1933 makes it an offence for an adult with parental responsibility to wilfully neglect the child in a manner that is likely to cause injury. This offence includes the failure to provide adequate medical aid. It was probably under this broadly defined offence that the police acted.

As a matter of law, criminal proceedings must be ongoing for a European arrest warrant to be issued. There must also be a realistic prospect of conviction. The first requirement does not seem to have been satisfied in this case. It is unclear whether the second was.

On 29th August 2014 Portsmouth Social Services successfully applied to the High Court to make Ashya a ward of court. The court now had control over all matters relating to Ashya's welfare and demanded that he be presented to the nearest hospital at once. The next day Ashya and his parents were found in Spain. Ashya appeared to have suffered no ill effects from his travels. His parents were transferred to prison pending extradition proceedings. This triggered a public backlash against the hospital and police.

On 2nd September the Crown Prosecution Service arranged for the discharge of the European arrest warrant on the basis of insufficient evidence for a realistic prospect of a criminal conviction. On 5th September the High Court allowed Ashya to undergo proton beam treatment in a clinic in Prague. Despite this, there were questions about whether the statutory authorities acted in a heavy-handed manner.

In a rapidly evolving situation the hospital and police were required to act quickly, without any clear knowledge of the intentions of Ashya's parents. The attempts to contact Ashya's parents after his disappearance were fruitless.

The law can be a blunt instrument, but without knowing what the authorities knew at the time of making their decision we must be slow to criticise their actions with the benefit of hindsight.

In terms of clinical ethics, the case highlights the interdependence of patient and family and the vital importance of clinicians and families working together towards the shared goal of doing what is best for the child. Although not infallible, mutually acceptable plans can – with time, negotiation, cultural and religious sensitivity, and a relationship of trust – almost always be found. The trick is to get the family on board early and to maintain regular contact, with opportunities for questions, so that the risk of misunderstandings, unrealistic expectations, and later opposition is reduced. Perhaps such 'preventive ethics' might have avoided the total loss of trust in Ashya's case.

Ashya had 30 sessions of proton beam therapy in Prague. Scans and tests conducted in 2015 showed the tumour had gone. He is now back at school.

THE CHARLIE GARD CASE – AN ETHICIST IN THE COURTROOM

The Charlie Gard case was another best interests case which captured the attention of the world for several months in mid 2017. Charlie was a beautiful little boy diagnosed with a rare inherited disease in September 2016. The question was whether it would be in his best interests to undergo experimental treatment in the United States. His parents believed it was. His medical team at Great Ormond Street Hospital, known as GOSH, disagreed.

As I passed the gates of the Royal Courts of Justice to observe the hearing in the High Court, the crowds outside were chanting "Shame on you, GOSH!" and holding photos of 11-month-old Charlie in intensive care.

In court, the barrister for the parents presented the new evidence in an effort to allow Charlie to undergo experimental nucleoside treatment abroad.

The parents pinned their hopes on a respected American doctor, a professor of neurology, who gave evidence via video-link. He had also given evidence in an earlier hearing in April.

In the doctor's opinion, which was based on his

team's recent, unpublished research not available in April, there was a 55% chance of the nucleoside therapy reducing the amount of time on a ventilator, and a 10% chance of complete weaning from the ventilator. The doctor was less optimistic on the impact of the treatment on brain function, but said there was a "small but significant chance" of improvement.

The fundamental medical issue, according to the doctor, was whether the brain was merely dysfunctional or whether there was irreversible structural damage. According to the doctor, the MRI and EEG did not answer that question.

As the American doctor had not examined Charlie, the judge asked if he would be prepared to come to London. He was.

The highlight of the parents' case came late in the day, when their counsel asked the doctor whether a clinical examination could resolve the dysfunction vs. structural damage question. No. "How then can we resolve this question?" asked the barrister, who surely knew the answer. "The only way to tell how much of the brain damage is irreversible is by trying the [nucleoside] therapy."

A key difficulty with the American doctor's evidence was that he never examined Charlie, or saw his medical notes, or all the imaging. He relied on summaries, reports and e-mails. He also said he would defer to the appropriate specialists in determining how much of Charlie's encephalopathy was attributable to a dysfunction or a structural brain problem.

After hearing the evidence, the judge told the lawyers that the American doctor was not, at present, sufficiently informed about Charlie's case to influence the court.

The outcome of the hearing was that a multi-disciplinary meeting would be held shortly, after which a decision would be made.

Counsel for the family said that any experimental treatment provided by the American doctor would have to comply with the Hippocratic oath. However, it is not clear that the oath supported the experimental treatment. The oath declares:

"Into as many houses as I may enter, I will go for the benefit of the ill".

The author of the *Art*, one of the Hippocratic essays, wrote: "I would define medicine as the complete removal of the distress of the sick, the alleviation of the more violent diseases."

The restoration of some muscular movement and some degree of cognitive improvement on a severely encephalopathic brain was arguably of no benefit. A greater degree of awareness and sentience could result in more, not less, distress, and more, not less, pain, whether physical or psychological. Cognitive improvement is no blessing if it falls short of the threshold of minimally acceptable cognitive function. The American doctor could not comment on the degree of improvement, but the preponderance of the evidence – and the earlier finding of the court – was that the nucleoside therapy was highly unlikely to confer any benefit to Charlie's massively damaged brain.

The hospital's rationale was closer to the spirit of the oath, as described in the hospital's position statement for the hearing:

"It has been and remains the unanimous view of all those caring for Charlie at Great Ormond Street that withdrawal of ventilation and palliative care are all that the hospital can offer him consistent with his welfare. That is because in the view of his treating team and all those from whom GOSH obtained second opinions, he has no quality of life and no real prospect of any quality of life."

If that was factually accurate, any aggressive care would not have been "for the benefit of the ill" and would have been contrary to the oath.

An important factor in this case was Charlie's current level of pain. Professor A, a leading expert in mitochondrial diseases, said in the earlier April hearing that Charlie was likely to have the conscious experience of pain. His treating clinicians believed in April that Charlie was suffering. The American doctor said at the hearing that he saw no evidence of pain, although he acknowledged that the tubes could be very uncomfortable. He deferred to intensive care experts. In intensive care, Charlie was on morphine.

If Charlie was in pain or distress, every passing day was a cruel one. The doctors were then in danger of violating another tenet of medical ethics: first do no harm. The experimental treatment would only have been justified if the harm of keeping him alive in intensive care and the risks and burdens of the treatment (which included the risk of cardiac arrhythmia and the prolongation, even worsening, of suffering) were outweighed by the chance of achieving a quality of life that was worth living. His current quality of life, all agreed, did not reach that threshold.

Shortly after the multi-disciplinary meeting and a new MRI scan, the parents announced that they were no longer seeking the experimental treatment. The US doctor saw the scan and withdrew the offer of the nucleoside therapy. Charlie was beyond help. He died on 28th July 2017, a few days before his first birthday.

The case produced no new law, but a unique feature of this tragic case was the role of social media and the Internet and the way a private decision became a most public affair. Donald Trump and the Pope were among the thousands who intervened in support of Charlie.

By judicious use of the Internet and social media, the parents challenged the medical opinion of the UK doctors by identifying dissenting clinicians from all over the world. They obtained funding for the potential treatment and, if it had been needed, the legal costs, removing a key counterargument about the use of scarce resources. They put enormous pressure on the hospital management, who would have been mightily worried about any damage to the hospital's reputation and a drop in donations. The hospital staff, lawyers and no doubt the judge were also under pressure and in receipt of threats and insults.

Among the deafening noise of the chants, the tweets and the posts, the insults and accusations, the ingenious tactics of the legal teams, and the concerns about reputation, the fundamental question should always remain: what is best for this sick child? As the distractions increase, so does the risk of forgetting this.

ALFIE EVANS AND GUERRILLA WARFARE

Less than a year after the death of Charlie Gard, another case involving a terminally ill baby dominated the front pages of newspapers. Alfie Evans, who was nearly 2 years old when he passed away on 28th April 2018, suffered from a severe and progressive neurodegenerative condition.

Alfie had been treated at Alder Hey Hospital in Liverpool from December 2016. As time passed, the relationship between Alfie's young parents and the medical team deteriorated, and the hospital trust eventually sought a court declaration to allow doctors to withdraw Alfie's ventilator.

In his High Court judgment of 11th April 2018, Mr Justice Hayden remarked that "almost the entirety of Alfie's brain [has] been eroded leaving only water and cerebral spinal fluid." The medical experts, including those instructed by the Evans family, agreed that Alfie's condition was untreatable.

Mr Justice Hayden held that continued ventilation was no longer in Alfie's best interests and declared as lawful the withdrawal of ventilation and the provision of palliative care. Transferring Alfie elsewhere was also deemed irreconcilable with his best interests.

171

Higher courts upheld that decision, rejecting legal arguments about the rights of the parents by stressing the paramountcy of the child's welfare and dismissing submissions of unlawful detention.

On 23rd April 2018, with all legal routes seemingly exhausted, 200 or so protesters turned up outside the hospital. At one point, dozens ran towards the main doors of the hospital only to be stopped by a row of policemen. As in the Charlie Gard case, outside the hospital and on social media, protesters hurled verbal abuse at medical staff: "kidnappers", "murderers", "executioners". On Twitter, thousands returned insults to the protesters: "ungrateful", "morons", "pathetic losers".

Although Alfie was a British citizen, under the jurisdiction of the High Court, the Italian government granted Alfie Italian citizenship that evening with a view, one assumes, to facilitate his transfer to Italy. The Pope had allegedly sent a military helicopter, complete with medical crew, to whisk Alfie away to the Bambino Gesù hospital in Rome. Alfie's lawyers lodged an emergency application hours later, which was dismissed by Mr Justice Hayden. Alfie had to stay.

The amount of judicial, police and NHS time spent dealing with this case ran to the thousands of hours. The NHS also had to pay its lawyers, including a Queen's Counsel, for the never-ending round of court hearings, depleting its limited resources by six-figure sums.

The whole situation, full of inflammatory language,

misinformation (how many commentators had actually read the judgments?), and delaying tactics, was profoundly distasteful. Hospital staff were terrified and so were the parents of other sick children in the hospital. In a new low, Alfie's father threatened to bring private prosecutions for conspiracy to murder against three of the treating doctors.

On the news, politicians talked dramatically of "state-sponsored euthanasia" and "judicial kidnapping", and drew comparisons with the Nazis.

Even in court, a usually sober forum for careful and measured argument, the judge criticised the parents' barrister for speaking "ridiculous emotive nonsense" and "using the court as a platform for platitudes and soundbites" instead of making proper legal submissions.

The worry is that this circus is becoming the norm in 'best interests' cases involving children, fuelled by social media and the public appetite for such stories. The creation, mainly through social media, of a maelstrom of opposition to the actions of the treating clinicians, with support from high-profile figures such as the Pope, celebrities, politicians, and even heads of state, has become a strategy to pressure hospitals into submission. It is guerrilla warfare. Alfie's Army against the NHS.

These guerrilla tactics do shed blood. The consequences, often, are that the children at the centre of the dispute receive burdensome treatment for longer than they should, treating hospital staff feel victimised and demoralised, and hospitals in the future will think twice about taking cases to court for fear of damage to their reputation even when continued treatment is contrary to the child's best interests.

Ideally, brewing disagreements between parents and paediatricians should be addressed early on, with unresolved cases escalating to meetings with a clinical ethicist or hospital ethics committee. Once the matter reaches court, the 'we are on the same side' stance is replaced with an adversarial one, with lawyers on each side. Hence why the courts should only be used as a last resort, when nothing but judicial intervention will resolve the disagreement.

After Alfie's death, some commentators suggested introducing mediation as a means to avoid legal disputes. It is a sensible idea, but the devil lies in the detail. At the moment, the precise form such mediation would take is not known. In any event, mediation requires the cooperation of both parties to succeed. In Alfie's case, independent mediation was offered but declined by the parents.

In the final pages of Saint-Exupéry's *The Little Prince*, the pilot narrator stranded in the desert senses that "something extraordinary was happening" to the Little Prince. He had to return to his star but was unable to carry his heavy body. Worried, the narrator refuses to leave the Little Prince alone. That night, the Little Prince walks away unnoticed. The narrator manages to catch up with him. The Little Prince takes his hand and says, "You will be sad. I will look dead but it won't be true…Here it is. Let me take a step alone." The narrator, full of grief, is unable to move. A snake with "good venom" bites the Little Prince's ankle, who stands still for a moment, without a sound, before falling softly like a tree onto the sand.

For months, Alfie's parents struggled to say goodbye to their Little Prince. They fought bitterly against it and can hardly be blamed for this. The parents' distress must be unimaginable. Yet babies like Alfie Evans and Charlie Gard, for whom continued treatment is no more than continued suffering, must be allowed to make that final journey in peace and dignity, away from the chaos of the outside word, the chanting crowds, and tweeting masses.

Alfie died in the early hours of Saturday 28th April 2018, 5 days after the withdrawal of ventilatory support.

BARIATRIC SURGERY AND JUSTICE IN AN IMPERFECT WORLD

"Dying granddad loses appeal for gastric band op" read one headline in July 2011. The dying granddad was Tom Condliff, 62. He was morbidly obese and had diabetes, renal failure, and various other co-morbidities. His deteriorating condition had left him depressed, incontinent, and unable to shower or dress himself. With a life expectancy of less than 12 months, he desperately needed to lose weight. Non-surgical attempts at weight loss – diet, lifestyle, and drug-based interventions – had failed. The remaining option, given his frail condition, was laparoscopic gastric by-pass surgery.

His primary care trust offered bariatric surgery, but a criterion for eligibility was a body mass index in excess of 50. Mr Condliff's was 43. As he was not eligible under the trust's general policy on bariatric surgery, his GP asked the PCT to consider him an exceptional case. The GP noted that Mr Condliff's misfortunes included confinement to a wheelchair and to his home, the inability to pursue his interests of attending church and playing the guitar, and being a considerable burden on his wife.

The trust was under a legal obligation to break even

at the end of each financial year. Legally prohibited from going over-budget, the trust had to balance the clinical effectiveness of treatments with cost considerations. The money withheld from one patient would be spent on another, bringing to mind a line from Samuel Beckett's *Waiting for Godot*: "The tears of the world are a constant quality. For each one who begins to weep, somewhere else another stops." Under these constraints, the trust rejected the GP's 'individual funding request'. Mr Condliff took the case to court.

The trust's policy on whether to treat a case as exceptional ignored social factors, such as age, gender, and parental status. Only clinical factors were considered. The rationale was threefold. Firstly, non-clinical factors, such as being married, cannot be readily assessed by the trust and could lead to subjective and unfair judgments. Secondly, if an exception was made in one case on non-clinical grounds, how could the trust know that other excluded patients would not qualify for treatment on such grounds? Finally, making decisions on the basis of non-clinical factors runs a risk of discrimination. The policy on individual funding requests gives an example: "If a treatment were provided differentially to patients who were carers this would tend to favour treatment for women over men." Such discrimination triggers a cacophony of legal and ethical alarm bells.

The court case did not concern the morality of the PCT's decision to withhold funding for Mr Condliff, but whether the PCT could lawfully refuse to consider non-clinical factors in its Individual Funding Request policy. Mr Condliff's barrister invoked a breach of article 8 of the European Convention of Human Rights, which states that "Everyone has the right to respect for his private and family life." By ignoring non-clinical factors, he argued, the PCT had failed to respect Mr Condliff's private and family life, a life whose quality was rapidly deteriorating for want of effective treatment. Further, he argued, the trust may have a duty not only to consider social factors, but to provide medical treatment under article 8.

No, said the Court of Appeal for England and Wales. The case law does not support the barrister's proposition which, in effect, would require the trust to favour some patients on social grounds. In his judgment, Lord Justice Coulson wrote: "The policy... is intentionally non-discriminatory." The trust is fulfilling its legal duty to provide healthcare within a context of limited financial resources. The policy itself shows no lack of respect for Mr Condliff's private and family life.

The decision in this case was consistent with the European Court of Human Rights' reluctance to meddle with agonising decisions on resource allocation. It allows the state a margin of discretion when pitting the interests of the individual (Mr Condliff) against those of the broader community (the current and future patients in the trust's catchment area).

In the concluding paragraphs of the judgment, Lord Justice Toulson rejected the argument that article 8 came into play in this case. Even if it did, he noted, the trust had "legitimate equality reasons" to adopt its policy. In other words, there would be a valid exception to justify the PCT's breach of article 8. As article 8 was a qualified, rather than an absolute, right, the state could interfere with it in certain circumstances, such as for the protection of the rights of others. This would have been one such circumstance.

The Court of Appeal did not, as some headlines suggest, make a moral judgment on the merits of Mr Condliff's case. No one disputed that his dire predicament was regrettable. The court merely dismissed his claim that the trust's policy, by refusing to consider non-clinical factors, was unlawful. In so doing, the court resisted an attempt to catapult human rights into the already contentious domain of resource allocation decisions in medicine. Primary care trusts will have breathed a collective sigh of relief.

The practical lesson for GPs, and patients, is to examine closely the criteria in the policy when deciding to seek an individual funding request. I can't help but wonder, however, whether the judges would have been swayed by more dramatic social factors. If Mr Condliff had been 35 years old, and the sole parent and financial provider for three young children, would the outcome have been the same?

Despite the court's decision, the trust agreed to pay for Mr Condliff's operation in late 2011.

THE CASE OF THE TATTOOED WOMAN

A 22-year-old woman presented to a district general hospital with an overdose of tramadol (a painkiller) and paroxetine (an antidepressant). She was morbidly obese with a body mass index of 51. She had been admitted to the hospital's accident and emergency department several times previously for deliberate self-harm and had required surgery to remove foreign bodies from her abdominal wall. After treatment for the overdose, the patient was discharged with community psychiatric follow-up. Roughly 30 minutes after discharge, while still in the hospital grounds, she poured lighter fluid over her head and neck and set herself alight. Spotted by nearby paramedics, she was readmitted with 15% mixed-depth burns to the head and neck. As the clinical signs suggested a serious airway injury, she was intubated, admitted to the intensive care unit for an overnight stay, and transferred to a regional burns centre the following day.

Upon admission to the burns unit, she had the burnt skin removed and a surgical tracheotomy. It was during the scrubbing and excision of the burnt skin that the theatre team spotted a tattoo under the dressings. In a prominent place on her chest, the tattoo read "DNR, do not resuscitate". No advance directive was found in the patient's notes. This unexpected discovery triggered a debate among the team in the operating room. After discussing the possible options, the team proceeded to initiate further resuscitative treatment on the grounds of 'best interests'. The rest of the patient's stay in intensive care was uneventful and she was eventually discharged to a psychiatric care facility.

No medical ethicist was available at the time of the decision, but the theatre team contacted me afterwards in search of a framework with which to analyse this and future cases and, to some extent, to validate their decision. What should the theatre team, suddenly faced with this ethical dilemma, have discussed?

I used the 'four quadrants method' discussed earlier to analyse the case and show how to put ethics into practice across a wide range of medical specialties. The approach, which can be used by doctors and non-doctors alike, consists of four broad topics or quadrants – medical indications, patient preferences, quality of life, and contextual features.

Medical indications

The first step in any clinical ethics analysis should be the easiest for doctors. It consists of reviewing the medical situation, identifying the clinical problems and the treatment options, and determining how the patient can be benefitted medically with minimum harm. It is particularly important to establish the goals of the proposed treatment and the probabilities of success.

Although the patient in this case had a difficult airway as a result of the burns, swelling, and a body mass index of 51, the medical indications were not in doubt. This was a young woman with reversible problems and a good prognosis. From a clinical perspective, she required urgent resuscitative care including invasive monitoring, ventilation, fluid resuscitation, skin debridements, and enteral feeding. The goals of treatment were cure, restoration of function, and prolongation of life, and the probability of success was high.

Patient preferences

The second quadrant puts in practice the principle of respect for autonomy. It focuses on the wishes, or presumed wishes, of the patient. In North America and the UK a competent patient is legally entitled to refuse medical treatment, even if it will result in death. Before asking what the patient wants, we need to establish if the patient is mentally capable of making an autonomous decision. If the patient is temporarily unconscious and urgent treatment is not necessary, it is advisable to wait until the patient regains consciousness and ask him or her directly about a proposed major intervention. It may be inconvenient for the staff, but such is the cost of taking the principle of respect for autonomy seriously.

Inconvenience aside, there are potential legal repercussions of failing to seek the patient's views. In the words of the former Master of the Rolls, Lord Donaldson: "It is trite law that in general a doctor is not entitled to treat a patient without the consent of someone who is authorised to give consent. If he does so, he will be liable in damages for trespass to the person and may be guilty of a criminal assault."

If time is of the essence, we can look for evidence of past wishes from advance directives, the accounts of relatives and friends, or the patient's GP. Many hospital teams overlook the possibility of contacting the GP, who often has relevant information.

In this case, there was no advance decision, at least not in the formal sense. Although the instruction in the tattoo was clear, the validity was uncertain. Was the tattoo done several years ago during a bout of acute depression? Was it done as a joke or a dare? Or was it inscribed during a moment of lucidity? There was considerable uncertainty about how closely the tattoo represented her current, deeply held wishes. In other circumstances, the team could have sought clarification of the patient's views from her relatives or GP but here immediate treatment was necessary to prevent further deterioration of the patient's condition.

Going to a shop to buy the lighter fluid and matches and inscribing a tattoo as an advance directive may suggest rational planning. The repeated attempts at self-harm may also indicate a consistent belief, but equally these facts could reveal an abnormality of mind. A finding of mental abnormality does not mean that we should automatically disregard the patient's views, but it does call for greater caution in interpreting those views. Setting yourself alight in hospital grounds, in close proximity to paramedics and medical care, may suggest a cry for help rather than a desire to die.

So, what are this patient's autonomous preferences? The answer must be that we do not know. The criminal standard of proof, "beyond reasonable doubt", is more appropriate in this context than the much lower civil standard of "on the balance of probabilities". A patient's life is at stake, and the risk of getting it wrong – of failing to resuscitate contrary to the patient's true wishes – is too high, the consequences too grave, to warrant the gamble.

Quality of life

The purpose of medicine is not merely to prolong life but to improve its quality. It is therefore essential to consider how a proposed intervention will affect the patient's quality of life. This is the task of the third quadrant. What physical, mental, and social deficits will the patient experience if the treatment works? Will the patient deem life to be desirable or will it be so grim that continued life will be a curse rather than a blessing?

There is a strong subjective component to quality of life and again uncertainty reigns. We cannot know how our patient will react after treatment. Will she be grateful for receiving another chance at life or will she be devastated at what she may perceive as a gross infringement on her liberty and autonomy?

Our evaluation of the quality of life of another person is subject to bias. Our beliefs about life and death, our general disposition and outlook, and our experiences all colour our judgment. We can to some extent dilute the bias by being aware of it and talking to colleagues whose biases may differ from our own. The solution, of course, is to ask the person concerned about his or her quality of life, but that is not always possible.

Under this quadrant, our medical team must again conclude that the patient has good prospects of returning to a state similar to the one she was in before the episode. Although she was evidently unhappy at the time of the suicide attempt, we cannot predict how she will perceive her quality of life after treatment or how this perception will evolve with time. This episode may be the trigger for a changed and better outlook. The team must therefore err on the side of caution and assume that treatment is indicated on quality of life grounds or, at least, not contraindicated.

Contextual factors

This final quadrant considers legal, cultural, familial, religious, economic, and other factors not captured by the other three sections. What does the law require? In the United Kingdom, when there is an imminent risk of serious harm and in the absence of a legally binding advance decision, it is lawful to resuscitate without consent if it is in the best interests of the patient. If best interests are unclear – and time permits – the hospital legal team could be consulted. The tattooed advance directive was not legally binding because it was not signed and witnessed. It was not verified by the patient's statement that it should apply even if life was at risk. In light of her psychiatric history, there was also reason to doubt her competence when she had the tattoo.

This quadrant is less defined than the others, setting the problem in a wider context. In emergency situations, it would be inappropriate or impractical to discuss some of these macro issues, such as the ethics of allocating scarce resources to treat patients who repeatedly attempt suicide.

Conclusion

In the cold light of day, this case may seem straightforward. Yet, at the time, under pressure, and with the patient's apparent wishes so plainly and strikingly inscribed on her body, doubt lingered. It will not always be possible to address all the issues raised by the four quadrants at the bedside, but even when time is short it should be possible to examine the key elements. The approach, like all other methods of which we are aware, will not always yield a clear-cut solution. The primary purposes are to provide a structured way of thinking about ethics in practice and to raise ethicolegal issues that may otherwise remain unexplored by clinicians acting in the heat of the moment.

In the present case, the positive clinical outlook, the reasonable uncertainty about the patient's true wishes, the potential for an improved quality of life in the future, and the clear legal position, strongly pointed in favour of resuscitation, despite the apparently contrary directions of the tattoo. Nevertheless, there is something troubling about the photograph of our patient unconscious on the operating table, with the tracheotomy and other external signs of aggressive resuscitation next to the tattoo's instructions. Situations such as this, where the head and the heart – at least initially – pull in opposite directions (the head towards resuscitation, the heart towards respecting the patient's apparent wishes) and where clinicians may disagree over the right course of action, are a good reason to use a structured method of analysis as a common starting point for discussion.

The use of a clear method is also consistent with the twin obligations to learn from experience by examining our decision-making and to share the stories and lessons with colleagues so that they too can learn.

The patient recovered uneventfully but continued to be depressed. She did not complain or display any anger about the intervention, nor did she express any gratitude. Two weeks after discharge, she died suddenly. The postmortem examination was inconclusive.

WHEN IS RESTRAINT JUSTIFIED?

Is it ever morally acceptable to restrain a patient?

A few years ago, I was the ethicist on a Ministry of Justice committee examining the use of a new restraint technique in young people in secure institutions. The committee was set up after *The Observer* ran a front page story detailing violent restraint techniques and the tragic deaths resulting from their use.

I was also, at the time, a member of a clinical ethics committee. In one meeting, the patient under discussion had severe learning difficulties and needed dialysis. Without it, she would die in weeks. The problem was that she became extremely distressed when undergoing dialysis. The clinicians decided that restraint would not be in her best interests.

In May 2010, a case was heard before the Court of Protection which raised similar questions. The patient was a 55-year-old woman who lacked capacity. She needed an operation to treat an endometrial cancer. Despite her fear of needles and hospitals, she had agreed to the operation in the past but consistently failed to turn up for treatment. The judge ruled that it would be appropriate, if persuasion failed, for a consultant anaesthetist to put some midazolam (a sedative) in her drink and to restrain her during the post-operative recovery period.

There are those for whom restraint is so repugnant a prospect that it should never be used. It is, they say, a violation of a person's autonomy and an infringement of their dignity.

Restraint is indeed a violation of a person's autonomy of action. The restrained individual cannot move even though he wants to. Often, it is also a violation of his autonomy of will, defined by Raanan Gillon as "the freedom to decide to do things on the basis of one's deliberations". Sometimes, however, the situation is more complicated. Did the 55-year-old patient with endometrial cancer want the operation or not? She agreed to it at first but when the moment of truth came she refused. Which of her incompatible views is the most deliberated – the agreement or the refusal? In Ulysses contracts, named after Ulysses' instructions to his crew not to untie him from the ship's mast come what may, the autonomous patient agrees to be restrained should he later refuse treatment. Restraining the patient thus becomes part of respecting autonomy.

Ulysses contracts are rare. Restraint usually requires the violation of autonomy. It can be violent and there is, inevitably, a risk of harm. In the 'nose distraction' technique, now no longer used in young offenders' institutions, the 'restrainer' strikes the child underneath the nose with the ridge of the hand. It is easy to get wrong. One could hit too hard or in the wrong place, causing a nose bleed, a broken nose, and psychological harm. This risk of harm must be justified. One justification is to protect others from harm.

The Observer article talks of using brutal techniques on "unruly children". Imagine a large, muscular, irate 17-year-old male, an improvised weapon in hand, fighting viciously with another boy. 'Unruly' is not the right word. It is easy to dismiss the use of restraints as barbaric and undignified, as remnants of the bad old days when it was undoubtedly abused, but such an outright dismissal ignores the realities on the ground. When a boy has his teeth embedded in another boy's neck, these arguments lose much of their appeal.

Another consideration is the risk of harm to the restrained individual. The risk of the restraint must be balanced with the risk of not restraining. One of the key roles of the Ministry of Justice committee was to identify and assess all the risks and harms, physical and psychological, of a new restraint technique. This also included an analysis of the potential harms on the restrainer. The nose distraction technique, for example, left the restrainer's hands perilously close to the young person's teeth. Only then can a proper evaluation of the pros and cons of restraint be made. In the case of the dialysis patient, the risk of non-restraint was an earlier death than if dialysis was imposed. The clinicians, however, deemed that the profound psychological harm of forced treatment, coupled with the practical difficulty of administering dialysis and enforcing adherence in between sessions, outweighed the benefit of a prolonged life.

Whether in a secure institution, a hospital, or in the community, the use of restraint should be a last resort. It *is* often barbaric and undignified. It generally does violate autonomy and cause harm, sometimes very serious harm. All practicable and less invasive alternatives, such as persuasion and de-escalation techniques, must have been exhausted. The restraint must be effective, its benefits must outweigh its harms, and those performing the technique must be adequately trained. Measures to deal with adverse outcomes must also be in place. In the endometrial cancer case, for example, the anaesthetist would need to anticipate the possibility of over-sedation and breathing difficulties. If appropriate, post-incident counselling should be offered to the restrained and the restrainer. The hard question is not 'is restraint ever appropriate?' but 'in what circumstances is it appropriate?'.

THE END OF LIFE

PAVING THE WAY FOR ASSISTED SUICIDE

On 10th December 2008, a controversial documentary showed the suicide of Craig Ewert, a 59-year-old man with motor neurone disease. We see Craig in an apartment in Zurich, surrounded by his wife and a social worker, switch off his time-controlled ventilator. Unable to press the switch with his fingers, he does so with his teeth. The social worker hands him a potion of sodium pentobarbital. "Mr Ewert," he says, "if you drink this you're going to die."

Craig sucks the liquid through a straw and grimaces. He asks for apple juice to wash away the unpleasant taste. At his request, the first movement of Beethoven's *Ninth Symphony* resounds around the room. "Thank you," he says after finishing the cocktail. The camera is fixed on Craig. Gradually his eyes close. He falls asleep.

The documentary, *Right to Die?*, follows two couples in their search for a peaceful death with the aid of the Swiss group Dignitas: Craig and Mary Ewert and George and Betty Coumbias. Unlike Craig, septuagenarian George was not terminally ill, nor in a wheelchair. He had had a series of heart attacks and lamented his inability to play tennis or golf or have sex. He wanted to die while still in relatively good health. His wife, although healthy, could not contemplate a life without him and wanted to die with her husband.

Although they loved their two adult children, they loved each other more and wanted to leave this world together. The founder of Dignitas, the human rights lawyer Ludwig Minelli, agreed to refer them to a doctor, a 75-year-old retired surgeon. He rejected their request for a lethal prescription.

The two couples engender quite different responses in the viewer (we know that Craig and Mary would give everything for the kind of life that George and Betty wanted to end), and the film's brilliance lies in the juxtaposition of the stories and the neutrality of the commentary, neither moralising nor facile in its approach to the issue. Although I don't think the programme presented new arguments for or against the practice of assisted suicide, the lived experiences of the couples did help me clarify my own views about it.

It is tempting to offer a noncommittal analysis: oh, aren't these heart-wrenching cases? Isn't assisted suicide a terribly difficult, multifaceted issue? Aren't the arguments for and against so evenly balanced? At the risk of drowning in an ocean of hate mail, let me show my cards: I believe that assisted suicide is not morally wrong and that, with appropriate safeguards, it should be decriminalised in the United Kingdom. John Zaritsky's documentary reinforced my belief in the moral permissibility of helping people die in exceptional circumstances.

Of course, good palliative care can alleviate most

types of pain; of course, assisted suicide must be a last resort after all reasonable alternatives have been considered; of course, procedural safeguards must be in place to avoid abuse and exploitation; of course, medicine is principally concerned with saving or prolonging life and not helping patients to die. But assisted suicide can, under some conditions, be consistent with all of these.

Palliative care is powerless in rare cases (and targets the physical pain, not the existential anguish); all alternatives may have been exhausted; procedures may be robust enough to indicate autonomous choice and unbearable suffering; and death can be a benefit rather than a harm to the suffering patient.

Although the documentary deepened my conviction in the moral rightness of individual acts of assisted suicide (on the basis of the twin ethical principles of respect for autonomy and beneficence), it raised serious concerns about the public policy allowing such acts to be performed. The footage did not inspire confidence in the current procedures for assisted suicide in Switzerland, exposing them as worryingly slack.

Candidates for assisted suicide are not always assessed by clinicians with the required professional expertise. A retired surgeon may not be the most appropriate person to assess the competence and suitability of candidates, and the danger is that rejected candidates will fish around for someone who will satisfy their request. I would not advocate such a system in Britain, much preferring the more demanding criteria of Oregon's Death with Dignity Act. Based on my sole viewing of the documentary, I thought the Dignitas experience seemed uncomfortably clandestine and amateurish.

Zaritsky's film is difficult to watch. The camera is unflinching, dwelling at length on the protagonists to capture the suffering etched in their faces. We are invited to transcend the boundary from public to private, seeing Mary shave and bathe Craig and following them both into the living room – or dying room – of the austere Zurich apartment where Craig bids his final farewell.

Some of the shots were reminiscent of scenes from Julian Schnabel's film *The Diving Bell and the Butterfly*, which follows the life of a man with locked-in syndrome. Only the stone-hearted will not feel moved by Craig and Mary's courage in the face of barely imaginable hardships. We must hope that such ills will not befall us and, should they do so, that we can confront them with equal courage.

Shortly before his death Craig composed an email message to his adult children in the United States. He wrote: "This is a journey that we all must make at some time. I would hope that this is not a cause of major distress to those who love me, and I expect that my dear sweet wife will have the greatest loss, as we have been together for 37 years in the deepest intimacy."

If I am unlucky enough to be in a situation where the final stretch is long and bumpy, I hope that we will by then have built a new road that is smooth and direct. I'm in no rush to complete the journey, but I would much prefer we started building this new road now. Oregon, California, Colorado, Belgium, Switzerland, Finland, and other jurisdictions, as well as people like Craig and Mary, all have helped to pave the way. We must not be afraid to complete it.

The failure to change the law in the high-profile 'right to die' cases of Tony Nicklinson, who had locked-in syndrome, in 2014, and Noel Conway, the retired lecturer who suffered from motor neurone disease, in 2017 suggests that it will be for Parliament, rather than the judiciary, to complete the paving.

ALLOWING NATURAL DEATH

In a scene from the film *Dumb and Dumber*, Lloyd Christmas, played by Jim Carrey, sees a fellow diner collapse in a restaurant. The man clutches his abdomen and complains of an ulcer. "It's OK," Christmas reassures the victim, "I know CPR." The man resists mouth-to-mouth. "It's a lot easier if you just lay back," Christmas notes.

While perhaps not quite as ignorant as the well-meaning Christmas, it is widely known that many non-clinicians hold rosy views about the nature and efficacy of cardiopulmonary resuscitation (CPR). Several studies have revealed their misplaced optimism: in one, the 269 respondents reported a mean expected survival rate for CPR of 65%; in another, 81% of respondents over 70 years old believed the likelihood of leaving the hospital following a cardiac arrest to be at least 50%. The real figure, for all in-hospital cardiac arrests, is roughly 14%, and many survivors will have new functional or neurological impairments.

The illusion of CPR's efficacy can lead patients and relatives to make ill-informed choices about end-of-life care. To stress the fallibility of the exercise, many institutions have abandoned the term 'Do Not

Resuscitate' (DNR) in favour of 'Do Not Attempt Resuscitation' (DNAR). Still, the discussion about the suitability of a DNAR order can be difficult for patients, relatives, and clinicians alike. So awkward can it be that many such discussions, which should form an important component of the future care plan, are avoided entirely.

Although raising the issue of death is seldom easy, part of the struggle is to dispel misunderstandings about DNR. DNR does not mean 'do not treat', much less 'do not bother'. With the exception of those in intensive care, many patients with DNR orders survive to discharge. DNR means 'if the patient has a cardiac arrest, do not start cardiopulmonary resuscitation'. Indeed, most trusts now use the acronym DNACPR. The manner in which the situation is described is arguably more important in resuscitation decisions, when tension, fear, and guilt may be palpable, than in any other area of medicine. To help dispel myths and improve understanding, a further change of terminology has been suggested: Allow Natural Death (AND).

A study published in 2009 on the views of nurses, nursing students, and laypersons in South Texas showed that changing the title from DNR to AND increased endorsement of the order in all three groups, reaching statistical significance in the latter two. It is not a surprising result, given AND's gentler, more benevolent tone. It is devoid of the cold negativity of 'do not resuscitate', with its connotations of patient abandonment and a death sentence. AND better reflects what so many of us believe should happen when the bell tolls: the peaceful, unobstructed flow from life to death.

Adopting the change should help reduce stress and feelings of guilt in all parties and may encourage clinicians to initiate the discussion with suitable patients or relatives more often than they currently do. The situation where patients who should have been DNR are resuscitated and, in a hopeless condition, left on the ward to die a second time should become less frequent. Not only will the indignity of CPR on the inexorably dying occur less often, but the finance managers, recognising the potential savings of fewer days on the ward, should rejoice at the likely cost implications of the change.

There are problems with AND, not least the potential for mistaking AND with the conjunction 'and'. In the early days of implementation, we should follow the example of one US institution which used AND/DNR to accustom staff to the new terminology. Once the new acronym is widely known and the DNR part can be dropped, we should find a way to distinguish AND from its more pedestrian homograph, perhaps by circling the term, or some other simple method.

AND lacks the specificity of DNAR or DNACPR. Allowing natural death, understood literally, may require withholding or withdrawing all sorts of treatment from the patient: no ventilation, no antibiotics, no dialysis, no palliation. Yet, often, it may be appropriate to treat a DNR patient therapeutically. If introduced, we must determine exactly what we mean by the term to avoid misinterpretation.

AND, like DNR, does not necessarily entail forgoing aggressive treatment, and admittedly this fact does not sit comfortably with the literal interpretation of 'Allow Natural Death'. As with DNAR, any discussion of AND would be accompanied by a discussion of what care should and should not be offered. The vagueness of AND, rather than being a disadvantage, could encourage clinicians to have that discussion with patients and relatives.

If a change of terminology can improve end-of-life care by reducing both anxiety and costs, then surely such change is morally desirable, if not perhaps morally obligatory. The immediate priority is to identify, as exhaustively as possible, the logistical and practical challenges of making the transition from DNAR to AND, and to address them.

We have much to learn from those pioneering institutions in the United States and the United Kingdom who have already effected the change. While changing the language alone will not overcome all the problems with resuscitation decisions, it is a step in the right direction, towards a healthier relationship between patients, relatives, and clinicians, and a more peaceful end for many.

CAUTIONARY TALES ABOUT DNACPR

Decisions about inappropriate DNACPR (Do not attempt cardiopulmonary resuscitation) orders continue to make headlines. Some will remember the landmark case of Janet Tracey, who was given a diagnosis of lung cancer in February 2011. A few weeks later she broke her neck in a road traffic crash and was admitted to Addenbrooke's Hospital in Cambridge. The Court of Appeal for England and Wales later found that the anaesthetist completed a DNACPR notice without discussing it with Mrs Tracey. This failure to involve the patient, the court held, breached article 8 of the European Convention on Human Rights – namely, the right to respect for private life (which includes respect for the patient's autonomy, integrity, dignity, and quality of life).

In a blog post published in August 2015 the solicitor from the firm Leigh Day, who had acted against the NHS in the Tracey case, reported receiving four or five queries a month about DNACPR decisions. She wrote, "Families leave me voicemails calling their loved one's doctor a murderer, such is the level of mistrust and suspicion aroused by finding a DNR [Do not resuscitate] decision has been made without prior information and consultation." Her conclusion was that the judgment in the Tracey case is often not followed and that "unlawful DNR decisions remain widespread."

Many years ago a consultant intensivist told me that she never used DNR orders because they caused an unwelcome shift in the attitude of clinicians. DNR does not stand for do not respond. As the US clinician and ethicist Joseph Fins observed, "a DNR order is simply a plan for the last fifteen minutes of a patient's life." It should not affect other aspects of care. The discussion about resuscitation is only one component of a broader discussion about advance care planning.

The main conclusion of the Tracey case is this: there should be a presumption in favour of involving patients in discussions about resuscitation unless there are convincing reasons otherwise. A clinician's belief that involving the patient will result in physical or psychological harm can constitute a convincing reason. The fact that a doctor considers cardiopulmonary resuscitation to be futile is not.

If the patient lacks capacity, clinicians should consult anyone engaged in caring for the person (or anyone who falls under section 4(7) of the Mental Capacity Act 2005) unless doing so is not "practicable or appropriate" or there is some other compelling reason not to consult.

Carl Winspear was a 28-year-old man with cerebral palsy, epilepsy, and other health problems. He lacked capacity in the days before his death on the evening of 3rd January 2011. He had been admitted to hospital the previous afternoon. At 3 am on the day of his death the cardiology registrar placed a DNACPR notice on his clinical record. He made the decision on clinical grounds and did not consult with the patient's mother. The medical note stated: "DNAR. Speak to family in the morning." In the morning Winspear's family contested the notice, and the DNACPR was revoked hours before his death.

The High Court held that a telephone call to Winspear's mother at 3 am, although inconvenient and undesirable, would have been practicable. The registrar's view that writing the DNACPR order was a clinical decision that did not require a discussion with the relatives reflected, in the court's view, a "misunderstanding as to the purpose of the consultation." The purpose, the judge wrote, was "to communicate the decision to the patient or in the event of incapacity... the patient's carer, so that important medical decisions about treatment are taken with relevant input into the decision making process, the principle of dignity and best interests is respected in the widest sense and the family can take on board and respond to the news." The court held that the hospital breached Mr Winspear's article 8 rights.

The names of Tracey and Winspear should echo in hospital corridors until the ethical and legal imperative of involving patients and relatives in DNACPR decisions is understood by all.

MEDICAL MISTAKES

THE HARDEST THING: ADMITTING ERROR

Even the best close-up magicians make mistakes. They are, simply, unavoidable. Good magicians therefore prepare for mistakes by rehearsing alternative endings and memorising quips in case of irreparable failure: "The real magician will be here in a minute," or "It worked fine in the magic shop." A friend of mine says, "At least if I make a mistake, no one dies."

Doctors cannot use that line. Their mistakes can lead to serious harm. While a magician's error is usually apparent to all, a doctor's error can be difficult to spot, especially by those who are not medically trained. The patient is, after all, already unwell by the time of the doctor's involvement. The first people who know that an error has occurred are usually the clinical team.

I remember speaking to a doctor who had been consulted by a couple with a severely disabled baby. On reading the medical notes, it dawned on her that the child had probably been subject to negligent treatment. The doctor nonetheless felt torn between her loyalty to her hospital colleagues and her desire to tell the truth to the couple. To my mind, this was not a moral dilemma. The doctor should have advised the couple to seek legal advice.

It is hard to overstate how much of a difference an award of damages could make to a family. It could cover the astronomical cost of care and allow the family to find suitable accommodation or modify their homes. I wondered why the doctors at the hospital had not revealed the mistake to the family. What happened during that morbidity and mortality meeting when the trainee presented the case to the department? Did no one speak up on behalf of the family? Did no one realise that silence might condemn the family to decades of bitter struggle?

Kroll and colleagues remarked in a 2008 study of junior doctors' accounts of errors that "we know remarkably little about the day-to-day management of medical error in the UK."

To find out more, the authors conducted interviews with 38 preregistration house officers. The authors identified a "strong sense of professional loyalty in which doctors, despite discomfort, kept quiet over others' errors." They also observed that "team feedback after error often prioritised reassurance: errors were normalised, dealt with through teasing, or minimised as being 'not the juniors' fault', 'not serious', or 'not a matter of life or death'. Deaths after an error were often framed in the context of inevitability: the patient wouldn't have made it anyway."

It is odd how doctors are reluctant to make prognostications in some contexts ("It's not possible to give an accurate prognosis") but quite willing to do so in others. In any event, it is not for the doctors to determine what would have happened in the absence of any error. As the source of the error, or close to it, they are at high risk of bias.

In another case a patient developed a swelling of the eye after endoscopic sinus surgery. A consultant assessed the patient and recommended conservative management. The eye got worse and, despite an urgent decompression procedure, the patient lost the sight in his eye. The patient was told that the blindness was caused by air in the orbit. A registrar carefully explained how the air had caused the damage to his optic nerve. The ophthalmic surgeons at the hospital published the case in a peer-reviewed journal, describing the cause of the injury as air in the orbit.

The patient eventually sued the hospital, which, remarkably, defended the case on the basis that the injury was caused by an infection rather than air in the orbit. The claim was settled in the patient's favour, although the hospital did not admit liability. As the lawyers involved in this case note, the trust's steadfast refusal to accept an error explains why "the public's faith in the medical profession's willingness to admit mistakes is somewhat jaded."

The GMC's *Good Medical Practice* at paragraph 30 states that doctors should be open and honest when things go wrong: "If a patient under your care has suffered harm or distress, you must act immediately to put matters right if that is possible. You should offer an apology and explain fully and promptly to the patient what has happened, and the likely short-term and long-term effects."

As of 1st April 2015, NHS Trusts (though not individual healthcare staff) are under a statutory obligation to inform patients if mistakes in their care have led to moderate or severe harm. This is called the 'Duty of Candour'. The failure to do so may constitute a criminal offence.

I will not tediously list the pros and cons of disclosure, nor will I dwell on the trite observation that admitting a mistake is painfully difficult for any self-respecting professional. In this situation, ethics has a right answer: forget loyalty to colleagues, forget the reputation of the department, forget about standing and promotion, forget about what the patient or relatives will think; the patient (or, if not mentally competent, his or her relatives) must know if a harmful error has occurred. The patient can then decide what to do.

There should be no more closing of the ranks. The interests of the wronged patient should trump those of the clinicians. And for those doctors who disagree, who are willing to let injured patients and relatives suffer without any compensation or explanation to lighten the burden, who are unable to put themselves in the shoes of the victim, I recommend an alternative career in magic.

PREPARING FOR WHEN THINGS GO WRONG

During his basic training as a fighter pilot, the astronaut Chris Hadfield was flying his jet in close formation, with jets immediately to his right and left, when he noticed a bee inside his helmet. Losing his cool would have endangered his life and those of his colleagues. Years later, in 2001, Hadfield was out on a space walk, holding on to the side of a spaceship travelling at more than 28,000 km an hour around the earth. He first lost his vision in one eye, and then the other. Again he kept calm. About 20 minutes later he recovered enough sight to complete the mission. He had been blinded by the anti-fog detergent used the evening before to clean his visor.

An even more perilous situation befell the Italian astronaut Luca Parmitano in July 2013. On a space walk Parmitano started feeling water on the back of his neck. The water gradually spread over his head into his ears, cutting off his ability to hear instructions, then into his eyes, blinding him, and into his nose, impeding his breathing. With considerable effort he managed to 'feel' his way back into the spaceship. NASA's report on the incident, which found that Parmitano's spacesuit had leaked up to 1.5 litres of water, noted that his "calm demeanor in the face of his helmet filling with water possibly saved his life."

In a TED talk in March 2014 Hadfield described his preparation for a space launch. He told the audience that in the first five shuttle launches the chances of a "catastrophic event" were one in nine. At the time of his launch in 1995 the odds of such an event were one in 35-40. He recounted mentally preparing for things going wrong during the launch, spotting which switches would need to be flicked for each eventuality. He then said, "In the astronaut business, we have a saying, which is: there is no problem so bad you can't make it worse."

The dictum applies in obvious ways to medicine. A surgeon reaches deep into the sylvian fissure of the brain in search of an unruptured aneurysm. Suddenly, it ruptures. The blood rushes up, flooding the operative site in high-pressure arterial blood. The temptation is to panic. Yet, a few seconds of hesitation could make the difference between life and death. One error can lead to another, making a bad situation even worse.

With his characteristic honesty the neurosurgeon Henry Marsh described in his book *Do No Harm* how he once used a faulty applicator when clipping a cerebral aneurysm. The fault could have led to a tear of the aneurysm and a catastrophic haemorrhage. Marsh was so frustrated by the situation that he shouted, swore, and eventually threw the instrument across the room. This response would not attract praise from the astronaut community.

The dictum applies as well to ethical issues in medicine. A poorly handled conversation with a patient's relative is left unresolved and escalates into a full-blown complaint. A medical error is deliberately withheld from a patient, only to surface later, with serious consequences for the doctor. The failure to respond appropriately to an initial problem will often confirm the truth of the dictum.

Like an astronaut, the well prepared doctor will foresee what may go wrong and rehearse an appropriate response. What to do if the aneurysm bursts prematurely, the needle enters the wrong space, or a relative disagrees with your proposed plan? In an interview in January 2016, Hadfield said, "In my experience things hardly ever go perfectly. Stuff goes wrong. That's just life. But we call that 'going wrong'. I think it's just 'going normal'."

DOING THE RIGHT THING

There are times when health professionals endanger their lives and limbs to care for their patients. Nearly 900 medical staff contracted Ebola virus disease in Sierra Leone, Liberia, and Guinea, with 513 deaths, in the Ebola outbreak of 2014-2015.

Army medical personnel have also risked all to treat injured soldiers on the battlefield, under the threat of snipers, ambushes, and roadside bombs. So too have the thousands of humanitarian health workers who have been victims of violence, or threats of violence, in conflict zones.

While physical courage is lauded by all, lesser known is the moral variant of courage. Moral courage is when you act on the conviction that something is morally right even though you believe that something of personal value may be lost. It need not be heroic in the grand, traditional sense. A doctor breaking bad news may show moral courage by avoiding the temptation to dodge the difficult issues. She will tackle head on the question about, say, whether the patient will ever walk again.

Since 2010, Washington Hospital Center in Washington, DC, has given moral courage awards to clinicians who have "exemplified the virtue of courage and acted against difficult and ethically challenging circumstances." A past winner of the award was a nurse, Crystal, who called a dying patient's family. The relatives were several hours away and the patient only minutes from death. Anticipating the inevitable, the medical team left the patient, but Crystal stayed behind. For several minutes she held the patient's hand and uttered comforting words. "No one should ever die alone," she told the colleague who eventually nominated her for the award. The colleague wrote, "We convince ourselves that we tried our best, so we move on to the next room while a patient dies in solitude. It is difficult to stand in a room and face what feels like defeat. So patients die alone because of our own cowardice and false sense that there must be somewhere more important for us to be at that moment."

In another act of moral courage a doctor may speak out against an ethical violation when all others are silent. At a morbidity and mortality meeting, the consultant orthopaedic surgeon describes how the operation was conducted on the wrong level of the spine. Another procedure, at the correct level, is needed. No one asks whether the patient has been informed, until a trainee surgeon raises his hand: "Has the patient been told about this?" In a hierarchical department where consultants are emperors, asking that simple question could require tremendous courage.

Under England's duty of candour, a health service body such as an NHS trust has a statutory obligation to notify patients of a safety incident that has resulted, or has the potential to result, in moderate or severe harm. As the organisation's representatives, doctors are responsible for discharging the duty. If their trust has not provided them with training or information on the duty of candour, they should ask for it.

And yet, even with the duty of candour and the GMC's guidance that doctors must be open and honest with patients, a culture of secrecy still lingers in many departments. In those places, a doctor who strives to act morally and legally will need moral courage.

At times, matters should be raised with those higher up the chain of command. Few doctors seem aware of paragraph 25 of the GMC's guidance on consent, which states, "If you think that limits on your ability to give patients the time or information they need is seriously compromising their ability to make an informed decision, you should raise your concerns with your employing or contracting authority." If there is no time to obtain proper consent, whether through lack of staff or some other systemic reason, doctors should tell the managers and include paragraph 25 in their letter.

Neither should long-term gaps in the rota be tolerated, which can push staff to the brink, violate the law on safe working times, and put patients at risk. The GMC states, "All doctors have a duty to raise concerns where they believe that patient safety or care is being compromised by the systems, policies and procedures in the organisations in which they work." Many doctors know that these practices are unsafe and probably illegal, but they do nothing. As Theodore Roosevelt said, "Knowing what's right doesn't mean much unless you do what's right."

Few doctors work in splendid isolation. Most form part of an organisation. The solution is to create an organisational culture where doing the right thing no longer requires moral courage. It should be expected, even encouraged. And if no award currently exists for 'moral courage shown by a clinician' in the United Kingdom, someone should create it.

WAKING UP TO THE EFFECTS OF FATIGUE
IN DOCTORS

On the evening of 12th February 2009, a Colgan Air aircraft carrying 45 passengers, 2 pilots, and 2 flight attendants stalled on approach to an airport in New York. The pilots failed to notice their low speed and did not respond to the stall warnings in time. The plane crashed, killing all on board. The pilots had travelled far to get to the departure airport and, in breach of company policy, had slept in the crew room the night before. The National Transportation Safety Board, in its accident report, concluded that pilot fatigue was a contributing factor to the crash.

Pilot fatigue is a recognised problem in the aviation industry, and there have been several symposiums on aviation fatigue. As a passenger, I am relieved that the industry is making efforts to identify the extent of the problem and to find solutions to reduce it. In medicine, the problem remains on the fringes. Some doctors will happily describe their struggle to stay awake on their drive home after a long shift, but little is said about the hours before, caring for patients in a similar state of somnolence.

Mention the European Working Time Directive

(EWTD) to a group of surgeons and a good many of them will pull faces of disgust. "When I was a houseman," one dinosaur will bellow, "we used to work most days and most nights, and we turned out all right." Others will nod in agreement. Then the old fellow will lament the advent of today's trainees: lazy, demanding, and quite unable to perform anything but the most basic of procedures.

And so, while some hospitals may be EWTD compliant, others tacitly encourage or turn a blind eye to violations of the EWTD. There are doctors out there who are working far more hours than the law permits and rotas that, under careful scrutiny, would leave trusts open to legal action. The true state of affairs on the working hours of doctors cannot be gleaned from a mere look at the documents. Until a case is brought, or some eagle-eyed journalist delves deeper into the issue, things are unlikely to change. The juniors are either too scared to speak out or have come to share the views of their seniors.

My focus here is not the EWTD, whose merits or demerits can be debated at length, but the problem of fatigue in doctors. In 2009 Matthew Worrall of the Royal College of Surgeons wrote: "There is much evidence that excessive fatigue leads to impaired reasoning and motor skills. But it seems there is a real lack of evidence for how that condition in an individual can translate into harm for patients in the hospital environment."

That last sentence brings to mind the illuminating 2003 study on the effectiveness of parachutes, published in the *BMJ*, which concluded as follows: "As with many interventions intended to prevent ill health, the effectiveness of parachutes has not been subjected to rigorous evaluation by using randomised controlled trials."

Fatigue adversely affects vigilance, alertness, motor coordination, information processing, and decision-making. These are qualities that, for most specialties, are essential.

There is no simple solution to the problem of fatigue, but the search for an answer cannot start in earnest until there is greater recognition of the effects of fatigue on patient care and physician wellbeing and an abandonment of the traditional, macho attitude of "to hell with sleep, just do it!". We are poor judges of our own tiredness.

In a 2007 study of junior doctors in New Zealand, based on 1,412 anonymous questionnaires, 30% of respondents had an Epworth sleepiness score greater than 10 (that is, 'excessively sleepy'), and 42% could recall a fatigue-related clinical error in the past 6 months. A 2012 report for the GMC on the impact of the EWTD concluded that, despite the beneficial impact of the directive, "trainees still work tiring, and potentially dangerous, working patterns."

The truth is that fatigue remains a problem in medicine. Change is needed at both the individual and organisational level. Reduced working hours may call for improvements to handovers at the end of shifts, for example. Individuals or managers may need to speak out against unsafe practices, be it about dangerous rotas, unreasonable requests to cover for absent colleagues, inadequate rest periods, manipulation of monitoring exercises, or even a belief that the next operation is one too many. In the face of anticipated opposition from senior colleagues or management, speaking out may require considerable moral courage.

Fatigue is not a sign of weakness or something that can be suppressed by a cup of coffee in the mess or a splash of water on the face. More research and education into the effects of fatigue on the performance and wellbeing of doctors are needed. Existing studies on the impact of reduced work hours on medical errors vary in their findings and their methodological quality. Research into fatigue, and the ways to manage it, is an area where medicine lags behind the aviation industry.

If the thought of a fatigued pilot at the controls of your plane is frightening, so too should be the thought of a fatigued doctor in a hospital or consultation room. Sully Sullenberger, who ditched his aircraft on the Hudson River in January 2009 after both his engines failed, noted that many of the lessons learnt by the aviation industry had been bought in blood. Ignoring the age old problem of fatigue among doctors will come at a similar price.

REFLECTIONS ON LAW,
MEDICINE AND MEDICAL ETHICS

SHOULD BOXING BE BANNED?

The British Medical Association's handbook *Medical Ethics Today* states unequivocally that "competent adult patients have the right to refuse any medical treatment, even if that refusal results in their permanent physical injury or death." Yet the BMA has for several years led calls to ban boxing and mixed martial arts on the grounds of the medical hazards posed to the fighters.

These two statements are difficult to reconcile. On the one hand the BMA says that we should respect Mr Smith's decision to refuse lifesaving antibiotics for his septicaemia but on the other that we should not respect Mr Smith's decision to step into a boxing ring against a consenting opponent. The consequence of not intervening in the first case is probable death; in the second, perhaps injury and a minuscule chance of death.

The principle of respect for autonomy forms a cornerstone of modern medical ethics. The principle requires, subject to limited exceptions, that people be allowed to make decisions about how they want to conduct their lives. This principle underpins the BMA's position that patients have a right to refuse treatment, a right that is itself anchored in the liberty principle, most clearly put by John Stuart Mill in *On Liberty* (1859): "The only purpose for which power can be rightfully exercised over any member of a civilised community, against his will, is to prevent harm to others. His own good, either physical or moral, is not a sufficient warrant."

For Mill, and for most democratic societies, this principle ensures that people can develop and flourish according to their own individuality. A democratic society thrives on this diversity. The liberty principle is entrenched in English law and embedded in many of the protections granted by the European Convention on Human Rights.

Why, then, should respect for autonomy, at work with Mr Smith the septicaemic patient, not apply to Mr Smith the boxer?

"The patient Smith harms only himself," you might reply, "whereas the boxer Smith harms himself and his opponent." This objection, however, is valid only if the opponent objects to stepping into the ring. Mr Smith's opponent benefits from the liberty principle as much as he does. Yet there are limits, in law and in ethics, to what individuals can consent to. I cannot lawfully consent to someone causing me grievous bodily harm, unless the activity falls within an exception, such as surgery, tattooing, and boxing. In its call to remove boxing and mixed martial arts from the list of exceptions, the BMA invokes the risk of medical harm.

There is little empirical evidence on the dangers of mixed martial arts, in part because the sport is relatively new. More evidence may exist on other combat sports, such as judo and karate. Since its inception in 1993, when rules and safety precautions were few, mixed martial arts has sought to protect competitors by requiring the wearing of gloves, gum shield, and protective cup under the shorts. Competitors are also required to undergo a range of medical tests, including magnetic resonance imaging, HIV and hepatitis tests, and an ophthalmic examination.

Contrary to common belief, the sport of mixed martial arts is not 'no holds barred' but contains 31 possible fouls, including head-butting, strikes to the groin, throat, and back of the head, and abusive language.

One study examined data from 635 mixed martial arts fights that took place in the state of Nevada between March 2002 and September 2007. It concluded that when regulated the sport has low rates of critical sports-related injury and that rates of acute injury are similar to those in other combat sports. Mixed martial arts bouts have fewer rounds than boxing, and the focus on the whole body rather than the head and torso means that blows to the head are likely to be rarer than in boxing. If medical harm alone is the issue, it is curious that the BMA does not call for a ban on other risky sports, such as skiing and taekwondo.

In 2007 I attended as part of a research project a mixed martial arts championship. To my oafish eyes it was skilful, fair, and entertaining (although as a traditionalist I prefer boxing under the Queensberry Rules). There was less blood on show than in many professional rugby matches. Still, I can appreciate why others may find it offensive. If we accept the liberty principle, however, offensiveness to some does not justify banning it for others. In a free society there should be a gulf between disapproval of an activity and banning it. Tut-tutters need not watch the fights. They do not take place in public places.

If studies show that mixed martial arts, boxing, or indeed any other sport is dangerous, doctors should emphasise the dangers, insist on safety precautions, and even discourage participation on medical grounds. We should be wary, however, of assuming that a person's best interests amount to no more than his or her medical best interests. How impoverished life would be – and how much slower human progress – if our desire for health conquered all other desires. Would Mount Everest have been scaled, the oceans' depths plumbed, or Antarctica explored?

Even if we concede the gravity of the physical harm of combat sports, it is Mr Smith who is normally best placed to decide whether the activity is, all things considered, in his best interests. The BMA's stance on this issue, which seeks to impose its own moral value on others, is at odds with its emphasis on respect for autonomy.

In the debate on the fighting arts, Mill's pithy statement is apposite: "Over himself, over his own body and mind, the individual is sovereign." At present this is a philosophical knockout. Further empirical studies could change the outcome. There are limits beyond which a civilised society should not go. If two goliaths stepped into an arena, even with consent, and fought with clubs until one was dead, the liberty principle would give way. But we are not there yet.

A PASSION FOR ACCURACY

When I was called to the bar, my father gave me a beautiful wooden box, within which were inscribed the words of Hardy Cross Dillard, once dean of the University of Virginia School of Law and later a judge at the International Court of Justice in the Hague. The text described the perfect lawyer, and one sentence read, "He is endowed alike with legal imagination and a passion for accuracy."

Even a cursory glance at people at the peak of their discipline reveals that a passion for accuracy, or attention to detail, binds them all. Although not enough to achieve success, it is a necessary component of it. The chess legend Gary Kasparov spent so much time analysing the games of his opponents before tournaments that a rumour emerged that he had a team of grandmasters conducting research on his behalf.

Michael Jordan was known in his pre-National Basketball Association days for spending more time practising on the basketball court than any of his peers. The elite group of 3-star Michelin chefs, though widely different in style, share an almost obsessive concern for perfection. It is a safe bet that all the medallists at the next Olympic Games, from archery to wrestling, will owe their triumph in part to a phenomenal attention to detail.

A passion for accuracy goes hand in hand with patience and persistence. Albert Einstein once said, "It's not that I'm so smart. It's just that I stay with problems longer." The challenge is staying focused for long periods when the task is dull. I can only imagine that studying the intricacies of the law of indirect tax is as soul sapping as studying the complex anatomy of the foot, but sadly there is no shortcut to mastering the subject. Patience and persistence require time, and a key concern with the reduction in doctors' working hours brought about by the European Working Time Directive is that they will no longer have the time to develop an eye for detail.

A passion for accuracy is also needed for the practice of medical ethics. In my teaching I tell students that good ethics starts with good facts. Although on occasion decisions cannot wait and must be made with limited information, most of the time there are opportunities to gather more facts and reduce the role of conjecture. In medicine, too, there are times when attention to detail is inappropriate. Harvey Cushing, the father of modern neurosurgery, was a slow and meticulous surgeon, but his precision was unhelpful when transposed to a busy military hospital in war-torn France.

The historian Michael Bliss compared Cushing at the casualty clearing station to a master chef working at McDonald's. Nevertheless, in normal circumstances attention to detail is beneficial. This is why it is risky for professionals, including doctors and lawyers, to give advice in so called 'kerbside' or corridor consultations. The account of the problem is likely to be one-sided and incomplete. The spectre of negligence looms ominously behind such requests.

In the United Kingdom professional medical ethicists are rare birds who seldom make decisions that directly affect patients. In recent years an increasing number of clinical ethics committees have appeared in UK hospitals. This is a welcome development. Yet, looking back on my days sitting on these committees, I am concerned that, although well meaning and able, our advice to clinicians was based on partial information. With luck, we would receive a short summary of the case, drafted by the requesting clinician, hours before the meeting. Occasionally the clinician would attend and briefly present the case. We never had the other side of the story, at least no more than the clinician's account of it, nor were we ever shown the patient's medical notes.

In such cases the risk of a biased presentation is significant. Deliberately or otherwise, the presentation may be structured in a way that favours the answer sought. There is no such thing as a neutral description of the facts of an ethical problem. What is said, and left unsaid, how it is told, in what order, by whom, what is emphasised and downplayed – all these affect the listener, even if only subliminally.

This unstructured approach is in contrast to that of the research ethics committee on which I sat, where we receive detailed protocols days in advance, spent hours reading over them, and prepared questions for the researcher. There is an uncomfortable asymmetry between the rigour expected of research ethics committees and clinical ethics committees, yet the advice of the second type can also, if acted on, affect patients.

What is the quality assurance of clinical ethics committees – or indeed of medical ethicists such as myself? Anyone reading this book could call him or herself a medical ethicist and set up a consultancy service.

If I were the chairman of a clinical ethics committee or a hospital manager, I would ask myself this question: if someone issued a claim in negligence against a recommendation of the committee, what would the forensic examination of the decision-making process reveal? Could we show a thorough attention to detail?

A passion for accuracy is not only a necessary element of great clinicians and committees: in each case it confers the added advantage of legal protection.

AN ESSENTIAL GUIDE TO MEDICAL NEGLIGENCE FOR DOCTORS, PATIENTS AND RELATIVES

One word that strikes fear in doctors is 'negligence'. When I visit hospitals in the United Kingdom, I enter safe in the knowledge that no patient will sue me, even if one collapsed before my eyes. I have no duty of care to patients, and without such a duty there can be no negligence. Doctors, however, have a duty of care to their patients, and hence it is unusual, in a clinical negligence case, for the issue to be in dispute.

Stepping outside the hospital, must doctors stop by the roadside to assist a person in distress or respond to the dreaded call, "Is there a doctor on the plane?" If they do assist, they acquire a duty of care. The person becomes their patient. But should they help in the first place?

This is where law and ethics part ways. In UK law a passing doctor has no legal obligation to assist a person in distress. However, the GMC's *Good Medical Practice* states: "In an emergency, wherever it arises, you must offer assistance, taking account of your own safety, your competence, and the availability of other options for care." Hence the non-assisting doctor may dodge the sharp horn of the law but still be impaled by that of the GMC. In this respect the GMC expects a higher standard of ethics than that required by the law.

Traditional medical ethics, in normal circumstances, would also condemn the doctor who ignored the call for help. In *Law and Ethics for Doctors* (1958), Stephen Hadfield affirms that "a doctor must give necessary treatment in an emergency unless he is assured that it can and will be given by another." The ethos of the physician is rooted in the benevolent desire to assist people in medical need. That is the raison d'être of the doctor. In the language of virtues, the doctor who ignores a cry for help may display selfishness and cowardice and lack the virtues of benevolence and compassion.

The existence of a duty of care is generally straightforward in the case of doctors and their patients, but what if the patient, through the doctor's negligence, injures a third party? A doctor may give negligent advice to a patient with an infectious disease, who then goes on to infect another. Or the doctor may deem a patient fit to drive, only to discover weeks later that the patient has had a seizure at the wheel and injured another driver. And what about the doctor who fails to section a psychiatric patient who proceeds to assault a passer-by? Can the victims sue the doctor (or, by virtue of 'vicarious liability', the doctor's employer)?

Several UK cases have shed light on the scope of the duty of care. In Goodwill v British Pregnancy Advisory Service, the defendants told a vasectomy patient that there was no need to use contraception. About 3 years later the patient began a sexual relationship with a woman. She fell pregnant, gave birth to a healthy girl, and sued the defendants for the expenses of the birth, the costs of bringing up her daughter, and the loss of income resulting from her reduced working hours. The Court of Appeal held that the defendants owed no duty of care to the woman. Lord Justice Gibson wrote: "The defendants were not in a sufficient or any special relationship with the plaintiff [that is, the woman]."

"At that time they had no knowledge of her, she was not an existing sexual partner of [the vasectomy patient] but was merely, like any other woman in the world, a potential future sexual partner of his, that is to say a member of an indeterminately large class of females who might have sexual relations with [the vasectomy patient] during his lifetime."

In Palmer v Tees Health Authority, doctors discharged a psychiatric patient who went on to murder a 4-year-old child. The child's mother sued the health authority on the grounds that those responsible for the murderer's care had failed to recognise and to act on the patient's real risk of harm to children. Again the Court of Appeal found that the health authority had no duty of care towards the murdered child, as there was insufficient proximity between the defendant and the child.

The test for the existence of a duty of care is found in the seminal case of Caparo v Dickman. It is summarised neatly by Lord Justice Steyn in Elguzouli-Daf v

Commissioner of Police of the Metropolis: "We must consider the ultimate question from three perspectives, namely (a) foreseeability of the harm that ensues, (b) the nature of the relationship between the parties, usually called the element of proximity, and (c) the question whether it is fair, just and reasonable that the law should impose a duty of care."

The test aims to keep the law of negligence within the bounds of reason. 'Fair', 'just', and 'reasonable' are hardly measurable, scientific notions. They involve value judgments. In my experience many medical students believe that the law, unlike ethics, always yields a clear answer. The cases on duty of care prove otherwise. The law can be just as messy as ethics, but at the end of the day judges must commit to a decision.

In 1954 John Bolam was a psychiatric patient at the now defunct Friern Hospital, London. To treat his depression the medical team administered electroconvulsive therapy, a relatively new treatment at the time. As they did not give Bolam a relaxant drug before the treatment, nor adequately restrain him during it, he sustained fractures of the pelvis. In his directions to the jury, the judge in a trial of the medical team stated the principle now widely known as the Bolam test: "A doctor is not guilty of negligence if he has acted in accordance with a practice accepted as proper by a responsible body of medical men skilled in that particular art."

After retiring for 40 minutes the jury found that the medical team had not been negligent.

The Bolam test applies not only to treatment but also to diagnosis.

Medical experts commonly disagree, but disagreement is not proof of negligence. The "responsible body of medical men" can be a small group, as long as it is responsible or reasonable. The key question that lawyers ask their medical experts is not, "What would you have done?" but "Would any reasonably competent doctor have acted in this way?" And in that question the relevant time is not now but the time when the act or omission took place. What is negligent today may not have been 10 years ago.

If the doctor is a specialist, then he or she must be judged by the standard of a reasonably competent specialist. The law does not expect excellence, merely competence. And for the junior doctors reading this, the expected standard of skill is that expected from someone holding your post in the hospital. As harsh as it may sound, no distinction is made between foundation year 1 doctors on their first day and those on their last day.

Doctors are often worried about making mistakes, but an error of judgment may not be negligent, even if it causes harm. The relevant question is, "Did the doctor in reaching this decision display such a lack of clinical judgment that no doctor exercising proper care and skill could have reached the same decision?"

Since its inception in the 1950s the Bolam test has come under fire from scholars. With the rise in patients' rights, some people have considered the test too deferential to the medical profession, too tolerant of views at the fringes of accepted practice, and too vague in its definition of a "responsible body" of medical opinion.

In Bolitho v City and Hackney Health Authority in 1998 the House of Lords modified the Bolam test. The court held that, in rare cases, a defendant will be found negligent even if a body of professional opinion supports the practice. When? If it can be "demonstrated that the professional opinion is not capable of withstanding logical analysis." The law adapted to the ethical climate by putting medical opinion under legal scrutiny.

The former lord chief justice of England and Wales Harry Woolf wrote in an article in 2001 that the expression "doctor knows best" should now be followed by the phrase "if he acts reasonably and logically and gets his facts right."

When I sat on a clinical ethics committee a few years ago we received occasional requests from clinicians who wanted to try novel procedures on desperately sick patients. I remember observing one operation in which the trauma surgeon, seeing that the patient was haemorrhaging uncontrollably, attempted a rare procedure he had read about in a case report the previous month. In such cases the issue is whether the clinician acted reasonably in the circumstances. In Hepworth v Kerr in 1995 an anaesthetist deliberately reduced a patient's blood pressure to provide the surgeon with a blood-free operating field. As a result the patient developed anterior spinal artery syndrome. The court held that the anaesthetist was negligent in exposing the patient to an unnecessary and foreseeable risk of major organ underperfusion.

In Waters v West Sussex Health Authority in 1995, however, a neurosurgeon who used a novel approach to correct a prolapsed thoracic disc was not found negligent, despite the patient's subsequent paraplegia. The surgeon had encountered a problem with the standard method and decided to alter his drilling angle, performing a laminectomy to relieve some pressure on the spinal cord. The court found that the surgeon did nothing that unreasonably increased the risk to the patient or that was contrary to reasonable professional opinion.

A solicitor once told me that he enjoyed clinical negligence because there were only 3 cases to remember and all of them started with the letter B. Two of those were Bolam and Bolitho. The third, Bailey, concerns the causation of harm, about which more later.

William Barnett was a nightwatchman at the Chelsea College of Science and Technology in London. On the morning of 1st January 1965 he and two colleagues had tea. Twenty minutes later they started to vomit. They drove to the nearby hospital, where they were seen by a nurse. The nurse spoke to a doctor on the phone, who advised the men to "go home and call in their own doctors." They left the hospital. A few hours later Barnett was rushed to the hospital and died from arsenic poisoning. His widow sued the hospital for negligence.

The court found that the doctor had failed in his duty of care. He should have examined the patient. Yet the claim failed because it could not be shown that Barnett would have survived even with proper care. The doctor was ethically culpable, but to establish negligence in law the widow had to prove, on the balance of probabilities, that the doctor's breach of duty caused her husband's death. In medicine this can prove challenging, as patients are often unwell even before they visit a doctor. Was it the doctor's negligence or the pre-existing condition that caused the damage?

No doubt the doctor in the Barnett case told himself what I have heard some doctors say after fatal mistakes: "The patient would have died anyway." This can lead to non-disclosure of the error. Prognostication, a highly fallible exercise one minute, suddenly becomes, in the doctor's mind, an exact science. Yet ethically it is wrong for the doctor who made the mistake to decide what would have occurred 'but for' the error. Not only might there be a lack of necessary expertise, but the doctor would hardly be an impartial judge. No one should be a judge of his own case. This is why there are lay people on the disciplinary panels of the GMC (and the bar disciplinary tribunals).

The doctor who justifies non-disclosure by saying that the patient would have died anyway falls foul of the GMC's *Duties of a Doctor*, which requires doctors to "be honest and open and act with integrity" and "never to abuse your patients' trust in you or the public's trust in the profession."

The doctor in the Barnett case, on hearing the nurse's account, could not believe that a cup of tea caused the vomiting. But what is causation? The complexities of causation were exposed in the impassioned debates on the link between smoking and cancer in the 1950s and beyond. It is only in the past 10-15 years that tobacco manufacturers have publicly admitted that smoking causes cancer and other diseases.

Philosophy has also grappled with causation. The editors of the *Oxford Handbook of Causation* note in their introduction that, in spite of the best efforts of philosophers, "there is still very little agreement on the most central question concerning causation: what is it?"

The law has developed an increasingly sophisticated – some say confusing – approach to causation, and causation arguments continue to appear before judges in the highest courts.

Readers may have heard of the 'but for' test of causation in law: would the injury have occurred 'but for' the defendant's breach of duty? If a GP fails to refer a patient in time, and that patient requires an amputation, a key question is whether a timely referral would have made any difference. This scenario would require an expert in general practice to establish whether the GP was negligent ("Would a reasonably competent GP have referred at that particular time?") and perhaps a separate orthopaedic expert to deal with the causation issue ("What would have been the patient's chances of avoiding an amputation if he had been referred by the GP on time?").

The law adopts a black and white approach to hypothetical scenarios. If the chances of an event occurring are more than 50%, then it would have happened. In Gregg v Scott, Dr Scott negligently assessed a cancerous lump as benign. As a result Mr Gregg's treatment for non-Hodgkin's lymphoma was delayed by 9 months. The cancer had spread, and his prospects of recovery dropped from 42% to 25%. The House of Lords ruled, controversially, that because the initial prospects were less than 50% the outcome would have been the same. He would not have survived either way. The claim failed on causation.

The 'but for' test was modified in the case of Bailey v Ministry of Defence. Ms Bailey was admitted to hospital for a gall stone operation. She was treated negligently during her postoperative stay at hospital, became extremely weak, and developed pancreatitis. The pancreatitis was unrelated to the negligent care. She was transferred to another hospital, where she aspirated on her vomit, had a cardiac arrest, and sustained brain damage. The judge found that the patient's extreme weakness, caused by the negligence of the first hospital, materially contributed to her inability to protect her airway from the vomit and to the subsequent hypoxic injury. This was sufficient to establish causation.

To recap, doctors cannot be liable in negligence unless (i) they have a duty of care to the patient, (ii) they have breached that duty, and (iii) the breach caused or materially contributed to the patient's injury.

THE JUDGE AS MEDICAL ETHICIST

D was 36 years old. He had a mental age of between 6 and 9 years and an IQ of 40. For the past 10 years he had enjoyed a loving relationship with a woman, P, who also had a learning disability.

In 2010, P became pregnant. The resulting child had such a disruptive effect on D and P that their relationship nearly fell apart. Neither parent was able to care for the child, and the council started care proceedings. So upset was D by the experience that he did not want any more children. In 2012, a court declared that D did not have the capacity to consent to sexual relations, and so D and P could meet only under supervision. This restriction led to a significant loss of independence for D.

To resolve the problem, D's parents considered the possibility of a vasectomy for D. The risk of chronic or severe scrotal pain from the vasectomy was 0.5%.

At the trial in July 2013 Mrs Justice Eleanor King, in the Court of Protection, was faced with this question: was it in D's best interests to have a vasectomy?

The court consulted experts and found that D did, in fact, have the capacity to consent to sex but lacked the capacity to consent to contraception.

The court looked at several factors. It held that D was capable of forming independent views. The court was satisfied that D did not want to have another child. The court also found that D was "broadly in favour of the idea" of a vasectomy, although in the most recent session he said he would prefer to use condoms.

The court considered the possibility of D using condoms. Despite extensive training, D still struggled to put on a condom. An expert advised that the risk of pregnancy over 12 months if D used condoms was 18%. The court concluded that D's use of a condom was "unreliable at best".

The court rejected the possibility of P, D's girlfriend, taking contraception, as she too was unreliable.

The court then turned its attention to the consequences of a further pregnancy. It examined the likely psychological distress to D but also to his parents. The judgment reads: "The court is not directly concerned with the interest of FG and JK [D's parents], but it is concerned at how their levels of tension and distress impact on D's welfare and comfort and it is clear that the impact is considerable."

Finally, the court looked at the effect on D's life if no vasectomy was performed. It held that, even though D had the capacity to consent to sex, D would still need to be closely supervised. This would not be in D's interests. The judge noted that "all those who care for D want to see his previous independence restored so that he can once again go to meet a friend for coffee or stroll in town with his friends."

The judgment then sets out the relevant law. As D lacks capacity to undergo a vasectomy, the court must act in his best interests. The court referred to the Mental Capacity Act 2005 and the requirement to consider all the relevant circumstances in determining best interests, as well as D's rights as enshrined in article 8 of the European Convention on Human Rights (that concerning the right to respect for private and family life).

The court identified a tension within article 8. On the one hand, if D had the vasectomy, he would lose his ability to decide to become a genetic parent in the future. On the other hand, D had a right to respect for his autonomy (such as it is), and that included his decision not to have any more children and to have a sexual relationship with P.

After referring to relevant case law, the court concluded that "the evidence unequivocally points to an improvement in the quality of D's life in the event that he has a vasectomy." The judge concluded her judgment by listing the factors in favour of the vasectomy and balancing them with the factors against, namely the slender risk of surgical complications and the operation's lack of protection against sexually transmitted infections.

It is, in my opinion, the ethically correct outcome, but the case struck me as having much pedagogical value in its careful, methodical, yet relatively succinct approach to the problem. The relevant background facts are presented in a manner that reflects the nuances of the case. So often, in medical ethics lectures or even in clinical ethics committees, the background facts are sparse. In my experience, most cases are factually messy.

The judgment examined the key factors in turn and supported its conclusions by reference to evidence. Too often, again, we rely on assumption rather than evidence. "What evidence do I have for this?" is a central question when conducting an ethical analysis.

In the judgment the relevant law, guidance, and precedents clarify the legal and ethical principles, and the balancing exercise of competing considerations is set out in a structured fashion.

It is unrealistic to expect students, clinicians, or members of the public to possess the analytic skills of High Court judges, but why not aspire to such clarity of thought and analysis?

When I studied medical ethics I was never asked to read entire judgments, merely extracts. I wish I had. Judges are the most pragmatic of ethicists, combining law and ethics to arrive at a concrete answer. They cannot sit on the fence. They shun the obscure language of ethical theory. There is much about practical decision-making that doctors, ethicists, and members of the public can learn from their judgments.

A GAME-CHANGER: THE NEW(ISH) LAW ON CONSENT

All doctors and patients should be aware of the landmark decision in Montgomery v Lanarkshire Health Board, given by the UK Supreme Court on 11th March 2015. And yet, when I asked 45 GPs in training if they had ever heard of the case at a lecture last week, only 10 said they had.

Nadine Montgomery was a woman with diabetes who gave birth by vaginal delivery. Her baby, Sam, was born with serious disabilities after shoulder dystocia during delivery. The doctor, Dina McLellan, did not tell Montgomery of the 9-10% risk of shoulder dystocia. McLellan said that she did not routinely discuss the risk of shoulder dystocia with women with diabetes for fear that, if told, such women would opt for a caesarean section. The court held that McLellan should have informed Montgomery of the risk and discussed with her the option of a caesarean section.

After the Montgomery case, the so-called Bolam test, which asks whether a doctor's conduct would be supported by a responsible body of medical opinion, no longer applies to the issue of consent. The law now requires a doctor to take "reasonable care to ensure that the patient is aware of any material risks involved in any recommended treatment, and of any reasonable alternative or variant treatments."

So, doctors must now ask themselves three questions:

1. Does the patient know about the material risks of the treatment I am proposing?
2. Does the patient know about reasonable alternatives to this treatment?
3. Have I taken reasonable care to ensure that the patient actually knows this?

To answer the first question doctors must form a view of what counts as a 'material risk'. The law defines it as either a risk to which a reasonable person in the patient's position would be likely to attach significance or a risk that a doctor knows – or should reasonably know – would probably be deemed of significance by this particular patient.

The focus on 'this particular patient' is key. A material risk to one patient may not be to another. A surgeon once told me that he discloses risks of 1% and more. This is a perilous habit. In the Australian case of Rogers v Whitaker there was a one in 14,000 chance of blindness in one eye. Although the risk was remote, the claimant was already blind in the other eye, making the risk of great significance to the claimant. The Australian court found the doctor's failure to disclose this risk to be negligent.

A pro forma approach to consent – repeating a memorised script – is a common but ethically and legally dubious practice. The UK Supreme Court talks of a 'dialogue' between doctor and patient.

The Supreme Court emphasised the need to give information in clear terms and to avoid "bombarding the patient with technical information which she cannot reasonably be expected to grasp."

If information is material, doctors should generally disclose it. They should not wait for the patient to ask for it. In the Montgomery case the Supreme Court noted that "there is something unreal about placing the onus of asking upon a patient who may not know that there is anything to ask about."

So, when obtaining consent, law-abiding doctors will ask themselves these questions:

1. Does the patient know about the material risks of the treatment I am proposing?
2. What sort of risks would a reasonable person in the patient's circumstances want to know?
3. What sorts of risks would this particular patient want to know?
4. Does the patient know about reasonable alternatives to this treatment?
5. Have I taken reasonable care to ensure that the patient actually knows all this?
6. Do any of the exceptions to my duty to disclose apply here?

To these six questions I would add a seventh: Have I properly documented my consent process?

There are 3 exceptions to the duty to disclose. Firstly, the patient might tell the doctor that he or she would prefer not to know the risks. Just as patients are not forced to read the instructions that accompany drugs, nor should they be forced to discuss risks that they would rather not know.

Secondly, the doctor might reasonably consider that telling the patient something would cause serious harm to the patient's health. Many years ago I used this scenario as part of my research on truth-telling in medicine: "Mr Smith is taken to hospital after a heart attack. He is recovering in intensive care, and his chances of a full recovery are good. On examination, doctors discover that Mr Smith has a form of cancer that is quite successfully treatable with modern drugs and radiotherapy. Mr Smith's father died from this type of cancer years before, and it is known that Mr Smith has a great fear of the disease. His blood pressure is in poor control, and minimising stress is medically desirable to lower the risks of another heart attack. Should the doctor, at this time, tell Mr Smith that he has a form of cancer?"

Three-quarters of my 85 doctor respondents answered "No." As long as the doctor's belief that disclosure would cause severe harm is reasonable, withholding the information will not be unlawful. The Supreme Court warns, however, that this "therapeutic exception" should not be abused.

Thirdly, no consent is needed in circumstances of necessity, such as when a patient in need of urgent treatment is unconscious or lacks capacity.

Ethically astute readers will note that the law now demands a standard of consent broadly similar to that required by the professional guidance of the GMC. Doctors who follow that guidance will not fall foul of the law.

Other readers will hold the view that consent is a myth invented by lawyers and ethicists and may ask, "How do we find the time to get such consent?" The court's answer is that the law must impose some obligations "so that even those doctors who have less skill or inclination for communication, or who are more hurried, are obliged to pause and engage in the discussion which the law requires."

The law is set. Some doctors will need to adapt. As Porgy sings, "No use complainin'."

WHO WILL OPERATE ON YOU?

Kathleen Jones had terrible back pain. Following the advice of Daniel Chan, a highly regarded and experienced spinal surgeon, in 2010 she agreed to undergo decompression surgery. She believed that Mr Chan would perform the operation and had waited for his return from leave so that he could undertake it.

Six days before the operation Mr Sundaram, a fellow in trauma and orthopaedics, asked for her consent to the procedure. She signed the consent form, which included the statement, "I understand that you cannot give me a guarantee that a particular person will perform the procedure. The person will, however, have appropriate experience."

On the morning of the operation a nurse told Ms Jones that Mr Chan was busy in clinic and that Mr Sundaram would be operating on her. By that time, she said, she was already in her surgical gown and believed that she had reached "the point of no return". The surgery went ahead.

During the operation Ms Jones sustained a large tear to the dura of the cauda equina that left her with significant disabilities. She sued the hospital trust on two grounds: that the operation was negligently performed, and that she had not given valid consent because of the late and unexpected change of surgeon.

The judge found that the operation was not conducted negligently but that the doctors had not obtained valid consent. They had infringed Ms Jones's "right to make an informed choice as to who would operate on her." The judge noted that "a decision [to consent to the operation] taken so far down the line is unlikely to be taken freely."

These findings are consistent with the GMC's guidance that doctors should give patients enough time to make a decision, as well as information about who will be "mainly responsible for and involved in their care and what their roles are."

The trust's lawyers argued that Jones would have been injured even if Mr Chan had done the operation. The judge disagreed, invoking the evidence of the neurosurgical expert instructed by Ms Jones that "experience counts". The expert observed that he now had fewer dural tears than in his earlier years. In short, if Mr Chan had conducted the operation, there would probably have been no dural tear and no injury.

The case, which was decided in September 2015, was heard in a county court and thus the decision has only persuasive (rather than binding) force in future cases. Yet it should give doctors food for thought.

Firstly, it emphasises the importance of making clear to the patient, in good time, the identity of the operating surgeon.

Secondly, it recognises that in operations where

"experience counts" the seniority and experience of the surgeon may affect the occurrence of complications. Is this something that ought to be disclosed to the patient? A close reading of the GMC guidance may suggest so: section 9(e) states that doctors must tell patients if the risks and benefits of an intervention "are affected by which organisation or doctor is chosen to provide care." Would this be practicable or desirable in all cases?

Finally, it shows that a signed consent form is not conclusive evidence of consent.

In light of the recent case law, the importance of doctors getting to grips with the requirements of consent cannot be overstated.

For us patients, we should not hesitate to ask questions from our clinicians about what they are proposing, including the alternatives, and to inform them of what is important to us, whether it's the identity of the surgeon or your daughter's wedding next week.

LISTENING TO PATIENTS IS NOT ENOUGH

A senior house officer working nights in an emergency department examines a 13-month-old girl shortly after 5 am. Over the past few days, the patient has had a raised temperature and vomited 3 times. She has passed urine and opened her bowels. She has no rash or diarrhoea, and she looks well. The diagnosis is an upper respiratory tract infection. The senior house officer discharges the patient.

Later that day, the girl's condition worsens, and she is readmitted to hospital. She is diagnosed with pneumococcal meningitis and suffers permanent brain damage. The parents sue the hospital trust.

The senior house officer did not record why the parents brought their daughter to hospital. The reason was that they noticed the child's eyes rolling, and this prompted them to call the out-of-hours service. The parents did not volunteer this information because they were not asked for it. At the trial, the judge accepted that the parents would have given the information if asked, and this would have led to a paediatric referral.

In court, the senior house officer said, "Usually, if [there are] rolling eyes, that is scary. I wouldn't need to ask the right question; the parents would tell me first

258

of all." The question for the judge was whether it was substandard practice for a senior house officer in this position not to obtain that information.

The judge found that an emergency medicine consultant or paediatrician would have elicited information about the eye-rolling episode, perhaps by asking, "This child looks fine to me, how was she different earlier?" But the judge said that a senior house officer could not be measured against the standard of an experienced clinician, and the case was dismissed.

The family appealed. The judge in the first trial had placed much weight on the trust's medical expert, who'd said that many parents attended emergency departments "without there being any direct and obvious precipitating factor." The Court of Appeal was unimpressed, saying "The fact that there is no clear precipitating factor in many cases is not an answer to a failure to elicit such a factor when there is one."

Asking parents why they brought their child into hospital was not beyond the competence of a senior house officer; if a consultant would have asked the question then so should the senior house officer. The Court of Appeal overturned the decision of the High Court, and the trust lost the case.

In short, the law expects history taking to be the same, whether it is by an inexperienced junior doctor or a senior consultant. Lord Justice Jackson said that history taking was a basic skill that hospital doctors at all levels should possess.

The senior house officer made two mistakes. Firstly,

thinking that the parents would offer clinically significant information without prompting; secondly, thinking that the reassuring history and examination obviated the need to ask why the child had been brought to hospital.

William Osler reportedly said, "Listen to the patient. He is telling you the diagnosis." This case shows that listening is not enough. You must also ask the right questions.

In an Oslerian vein, and no doubt aware of the crisis in morale among junior doctors, Lord Justice Jackson ended the judgment with an uplifting message: "Even good and conscientious doctors may, from time to time, fall short. That is not a reason to lose heart or (even worse) to abandon medical practice. Those who have learnt from past mistakes often have even more to offer."

LESSONS FROM THE FRONT LINE

In the summer of 2002 I was sitting in an Oxford café with a professor of medical ethics. I had just finished a masters degree in the history of medicine and, intrigued by the dubious conduct of some doctors in the past, was contemplating a career in medical ethics. "What do you want to do?" asked the professor. "I want to help doctors," I replied. And so started my journey in medical ethics.

Sixteen years later, now working as a barrister, I sue doctors.

The way to reconcile these 2 facts is that lawsuits, though miserable affairs, can lead to better, safer practice. But this only occurs if lessons are learnt. Here are further reflections from the past 2 months.

I represented a medical student in a fitness to practise hearing. The chief concern was his lack of insight into his rudeness towards others. Insight is a nebulous concept, but it can be broadly defined as the ability to understand intellectually and emotionally why a behaviour is wrong. Without this ability, learning is stifled and poor practice goes unchecked. A compulsory question for interview panels, whether they are selecting medical students or consultants, should be: does this person have insight?

On occasion I advise on cosmetic surgery cases. I attended a course on the topic last month, in which the case study, a fictitious one blending the stories of several patients, was a schoolteacher who underwent breast augmentation.

During the operation a nurse dropped one of the implants on the floor and, with no spare implant available, the surgeon decided to insert two larger ones. The operation was a success, but the patient was distraught. So obvious was the change that she became the butt of teenage jokes at her school, fell into depression, and quit.

Coincidentally, the next week I received a new case involving a patient who underwent a knee replacement operation. She was allergic to nickel and had asked for a nickel-free product. In the operation the surgeon removed the old knee, opened the packet for the new knee, and to his horror discovered that it contained nickel. Faced with a large defect cavity, he thought he had no choice but to implant the knee. The patient developed complications.

The lessons: do not skip or rush through surgical checklists. Remember that if the patient consents to one thing (a certain cup size or a nickel-free knee) you should not do something else unless there is a medical emergency and asking the patient is impossible. In short, do not stray beyond the scope of the original consent.

In the knee case the surgeon said nothing about the mishap to the patient until she asked some weeks later. She was distraught and lost faith in the surgeon. The lesson: be honest when you make a mistake, however daunting the prospect. You will be surprised how often patients forgive. Remember also the legal duty of candour.

Finally, last weekend I had the misfortune of attending an emergency walk-in centre with an eye problem. Sitting there, I witnessed the depressing sight of sick and injured people walking in, some propped up against a worried helper, others with bloodied tissues packed into their noses, and others pale as ghosts. They looked so despondent that the very experience sunk my spirits. When my turn came, the doctor was cheerful, diagnosed conjunctivitis in an instant, and prescribed some eye drops. I can now see perfectly. The lesson, all too easily forgotten in these litigious times: medicine is a noble vocation admired and appreciated by all, including clinical negligence lawyers and other wicked folk.

A CALL FOR CLINICAL ETHICISTS

In a 2005 editorial in the *BMJ*, I called for the use of clinical ethicists in UK hospitals. These are professionals, trained in medical ethics and law, who provide ethics support and education to clinicians and, in some cases, patients and relatives. Available at a moment's notice, they help prevent and resolve ethical dilemmas at the coalface. Clinical ethicists are common in large hospitals in North America and some parts of Europe but virtually non-existent in the United Kingdom.

Much has changed since the publication of my original article. The number of complaints against doctors to the GMC rose from 5,168 in 2007 to 10,347 in 2012. The number of new legal claims has nearly doubled from 5,697 in 2005-2006 to 10,686 in 2016-2017. The annual cost of NHS clinical negligence litigation has gone from £560 million in 2005-2006 to £1,707 million in 2016-2017. That last figure represents 1.6% of that year's budget for NHS England.

The morale of doctors has hit rock bottom following the conviction for gross negligence manslaughter of Dr Bawa-Garba, a paediatrician whose actions led to the premature death of a 6-year-old boy from sepsis (she was sentenced to 2 years imprisonment, suspended for 2 years), and her subsequent erasure from the register in January 2018 (which, at the time of writing, is under appeal). Many doctors felt that insufficient weight had been placed on the deplorable working conditions under which Dr Bawa-Garba was working at the time, which included her having to cover the jobs of absent doctors with a broken hospital IT system and a consultant who was teaching off-site. More than ever, doctors feel vulnerable to criticism and legal claims, let down by hospital management, and unsupported by their own regulator.

A steady stream of high-profile cases, most famously Charlie Gard and Alfie Evans, has exposed the complexities of ethical decision-making in practice, as well as the enormous public interest and scrutiny in the outcome of some of these decisions.

In 2013 the Francis report uncovered appalling deficiencies in care and ethics at the Mid Staffordshire NHS Foundation Trust, leading to the neglect and preventable death of hundreds of patients. Recommendation 215 of the report was the development of a common code of ethics, standards, and conduct for senior healthcare leaders and managers.

It is now trite to say that ethics permeates much of what clinicians do. The first UK journal devoted to the subject, *Clinical Ethics*, was launched in March 2006. My regular lecture 'tours' of UK hospitals reveal an incessant stream of ethical problems faced by clinicians of all specialties, including those not traditionally associated with ethical quandaries, such as pathologists, radiologists, and dermatologists. Yet, unlike junior barristers, clinicians have no obligation to attend any ethics training after they have qualified.

Sheila McLean, Professor Emerita of Law and Ethics in Medicine at the University of Glasgow, concluded in 2009 that "ethical decision-making in the UK is essentially ad hoc, and arguably lacking either in sufficient ethical expertise or in attention to legal process. It is also clear that CECs [clinical ethics committees, of which there are currently about 85 in the UK] are probably not routinely used by the majority of healthcare professionals."

In a 2009 study of 30 CECs in the UK, over half had considered fewer than 3 'live' cases (for which the key ethical decisions had not yet been made) in the preceding year. It remains my view that clinical ethicists are better suited to the task of providing support to clinicians than the often intimidating, impersonal CECs. An individual can build trust and form relationships with the medical team, patients, and relatives in a way that a committee cannot.

Since I migrated from the hushed halls of academe to the gritty world of law, I regularly see disputes that might have been averted by an ethics consultation or a timely lecture on the topic. Informed consent and best interest cases spring to mind.

Introducing clinical ethicists is not a panacea. The early recognition of ethical problems will not prevent difficulties from arising, and even the most accomplished ethicist cannot eradicate complaints and lawsuits.

However, common sense and experience suggest that organisations would benefit from having an employee with a detailed understanding of ethics, law, and conflict management, who can detect the signs of a looming ethical crisis in its infancy, and who can update and assist busy clinicians on ethicolegal issues in a weekly meeting or before a ward round.

The moral, legal, educational, and financial arguments for clinical ethicists are stronger than ever, as I hope this book has shown. Medicine in the 21st century is morally more complex than it ever has been. It is high time for an innovative trust or a private hospital to trial the introduction of full-time clinical ethicists – already tried and tested in the United States and elsewhere – and assess their value so that others can benefit.

At the very least, the appointment of a clinical ethicist would send a positive message to patients, relatives, and hospital staff that ethics is not an abstract buzzword but that it lies at the heart of high-quality care and that immediate, personal, and professional support is only a bleep away.

GLOSSARY

Anastomosis
> The surgical connection between two structures, usually tubular ones (e.g., blood vessels or intestine)

Anencephalic
> A birth defect in which a baby is born with part or all of the brain and skull missing

Aneurysm
> A bulge in the wall of a blood vessel which, if leaking or ruptured, can be fatal

Babinski's reflex
> A reflex in which the big toe of the foot is extended after the sole of the foot is stroked with a blunt instrument. The test usually forms part of a neurological examination

Bioethicist
> A person who studies ethical issues in medicine, biology, and biotechnology

Cerebrospinal fluid
> Clear fluid that surrounds the brain and spinal cord and protects those structures from injury

Cholecystectomy
> Surgical removal of the gallbladder

Decompressive craniectomy

A procedure used by neurosurgeons in which part of the skull is removed to allow a swelling brain to expand

Diaphragmatic hernia

A defect or hole in the diaphragm through which abdominal organs protrude into the chest cavity near the lungs

Encephalopathy

Disease, damage, or malfunction of the brain

Excision

Surgical removal by cutting

Exophthalmic goitre

A condition in which the thyroid gland malfunctions due to excess secretion of the thyroid hormone and the patient's eyes protrude

Factitious disorder

A mental disorder in which a person deceives others by appearing sick, by intentionally getting sick, or by injuring him or herself

Fasciculation

A brief contraction of muscle fibres causing the skin to twitch or flicker

Fibroma

Typically a benign tumour made up of fibrous or connective tissue. An ossifying fibroma is a benign bone lesion

Iliac fossa

The large concave surface on the inside surface of the ilium, one of the bones that make up the hip

Ilizarov method

An orthopaedic technique in which a fixation frame is used to lengthen or correct deformities and fractures in the bone

Intubate

The insertion of a plastic tube into the windpipe to maintain the airway open

Laminectomy

An operation in which the lamina, part of the bone making up the vertebra in the spine, is removed to relieve pressure on the spinal cord or nerves

Leukaemia

Cancer of the blood cells. Acute leukaemia, unlike chronic leukaemia, is a fast-growing cancer

Lumbar puncture

A procedure in which a needle is inserted into the lower part of the spine and cerebrospinal fluid is removed

Neurobiological

Relating to the anatomy, physiology, and pathology of the nervous system, which includes the brain

Oropharynx

Part of the throat, at the back of the mouth, which includes the back part of the tongue, the soft palate above, the tonsils, and the side and back walls of the throat

Pulmonary embolism

A blocked artery in the lung, usually as a result of a blood clot

Seropositive

A positive reaction to a blood test, usually one testing for antibodies and hence an infection

Sylvian fissure

A deep fissure in the brain, separating the temporal lobe from the parietal and frontal lobes

Tracheotomy

A surgical procedure in which an incision is made to the front of the throat into the windpipe. A tube is then inserted into the windpipe

Underperfusion

When insufficient oxygen reaches the tissues. This may cause damage or death of the tissues

REFERENCES

The chapters in the book were first published in various outlets. Most have been updated or modified. References to the original publications are listed below.

THE HARMS OF MEDICOPLASTY
  BMJ 2008;337:a1983
MAKE THE CARE OF YOUR PATIENT YOUR FIRST CONCERN
  BMJ 2011;342:d646
BEWARE THE LIES OF PATIENTS
  BMJ 2014;348:g382
THE LIMITS OF CONFIDENTIALITY
  BMJ 2017;356:j1505
DON'T FORGET THE RELATIVES
  BMJ 2014;349:g7351
HIPPOCRATES, MICHAEL JACKSON AND MEDICAL ETHICS
BMJ 2009;339:b3535
  "The case of Chelsea's Eva Carneiro shows how hard it is to be a sport doctor", *Daily Telegraph*, 18th August 2015
HOW (NOT) TO BE A GOOD PATIENT
  BMJ 2004;328:471

PATIENTS WE DON'T LIKE

BMJ 2013;346:f3956

A VOYAGE TO INDIA

"Indian patients suffer in silence", BBC News Online, 23rd July 2007

"India poses huge health challenges", BBC News Online, 6th August 2007

"It's tough at the sharp end of medicine", BBC News Online, 13th August 2007

HOW TO TREAT A PIRAHÃ: MEDICAL ETHICS AND CULTURAL DIFFERENCE

BMJ 2015;350:h850

New WHO safe and dignified burial protocol: http://www.who.int/mediacentre/news/notes/2014/ebola-burial-protocol/en/ (last accessed 7th April 2018)

DOCTORS AND TORTURE IN IRAQ

"Brought to heal or heel?", BBC News Online, 31st August 2004

"Do no harm": when doctors torture, *The Atlantic*, 12th December 2014

Ahalt, C. "Examining the role of healthcare professionals in the use of solitary confinement" *BMJ* 2017;359:j4657

THE MEDICAL ETHICS OF THE BATTLEFIELD

BMJ 2011;343:d3877

"The doctors' ethical dilemma", 11th March 2005, with Dr Kerry Bowman

AN ETHICIST IN THE NEUROLOGY

THE MOMENT OF TRUTH
BMJ 2010;340:c1992
HOW TO THINK LIKE AN ETHICIST
BMJ 2010;340:c3256
BATTLING PROFESSOR PINKER
"Guest post: the moral imperative for bioethics", Practical Ethics Blog, 3rd August 2015: http://blog.practicalethics.ox.ac.uk/2015/08/guest-post-the-moral-imperative-for-bioethics/
ON MORAL VISION
BMJ 2008;337:a1562
THE SLIPPERINESS OF FUTILITY
BMJ 2009;338:b2222
CLARIFYING BEST INTERESTS
BMJ 2008;337:a994
EMBRACING THE ETHICALLY COMPLICATED PATIENT
BMJ 2016;354:i3727
LESSONS FROM THE ASHYA KING CASE
BMJ 2014;349:g5563, with Aidan O'Brian
THE CHARLIE GARD CASE – AN ETHICIST IN THE COURTROOM
BMJ Opinion, 14th July 2017
ALFIE EVANS AND GUERRILLA WARFARE
BMJ Opinion, 24th April 2018
BARIATRIC SURGERY AND JUSTICE IN AN IMPERFECT WORLD
BMJ 2011; 343:d4944
THE CASE OF THE TATTOOED WOMAN
BMJ 2011;343:d5528

WHEN IS RESTRAINT JUSTIFIED?
BMJ 2010;341:C4147

Townsend, M. "Revealed: brutal guide to punishing jailed youths." *The Observer*, 18th July 2010 (http://www.guardian.co.uk/society/2010/jul/18/guide-punishing-jailed-youths).

DH NHS Foundation Trust v PS [2010] EWHC 1217

PAVING THE WAY FOR ASSISTED SUICIDE
BMJ 2008;337:a3010

ALLOWING NATURAL DEATH
BMJ 2009;338:b1723

CAUTIONARY TALES ABOUT DNACPR
BMJ 2016;352:i26

THE HARDEST THING: ADMITTING ERROR
BMJ 2012;344:e3085

PREPARING FOR WHEN THINGS GO WRONG
BMJ 2016;354:i4627

DOING THE RIGHT THING
BMJ 2015;351:h5288

WAKING UP TO THE EFFECTS OF FATIGUE IN DOCTORS
BMJ 2013;347:f4906

SHOULD BOXING BE BANNED?
BMJ 2011;343:d6937

A PASSION FOR ACCURACY
BMJ 2012;345:e4977

AN ESSENTIAL GUIDE TO MEDICAL

NEGLIGENCE FOR DOCTORS, PATIENTS, AND RELATIVES

BMJ 2012;345:e6804

BMJ 2012;345:e7858

BMJ 2013;346:f285

THE JUDGE AS MEDICAL ETHICIST

BMJ 2013;347:f5299

A GAME-CHANGER: THE NEW(ISH) LAW ON CONSENT

BMJ 2015;350:h1481

WHO WILL OPERATE ON YOU?

BMJ 2016;355:i5447

LISTENING TO PATIENTS IS NOT ENOUGH

BMJ 2017;357:j2670

LESSONS FROM THE FRONT LINE

BMJ 2017;359:j4624

A CALL FOR CLINICAL ETHICISTS

BMJ 2014;349:g5342